STOP
THE WORLDS CHRONIC KILLERS

STOP
THE WORLDS CHRONIC KILLERS
AND LOOK YOUTHFUL, HEALTHIER ON YOUR WAY TOWARDS 100

Tim Ekwulugo
and Teamlink Pharmaceuticals Ltd

authorHOUSE®

AuthorHouse™
1663 Liberty Drive
Bloomington, IN 47403
www.authorhouse.com
Phone: 1-800-839-8640

Published by AuthorHouse   12/14/2012

ISBN: 978-1-4772-4607-8 (sc)
ISBN: 978-1-4772-4608-5 (e)

TABLE OF CONTENTS

Introduction..v

Chapter 1

1.00   Good health and good living...1

1.10   Common killers of good looks and good health 3

1.20   Its always better to start reasonably early 6

1.30   Prevention is always better than cure....................................7

1.40   Its never too late to say yes to change..................................9

1.50   You are what you eat...11

1.60   Healthy life style that can lead to longevity.........................12

1.70   Foods that burn fats...15

Chapter 2

2.00   Diets...18

2.10   Choosing your daily diet..19

2.20   Balanced diet..20

2.30   Designing a balanced diet..22

2.40   Calories...25

2.50   Calorie dense food...27

2.60   Nutrients and Essential nutrients...29

2.70   Nutrients dense foods..31

2.80   Antioxidants...33

2.90   Enzymes...35

Chapter 3

3.00   Fats...38

3.10   Bad fats 39

3.20   Good Fats...40

3.30   Low fat foods 44

3.40   High fat foods 46

3.50   Reducing blood cholesterol and fats 48

3.60   Bad and good foods 52

3.70   Foods that make you look older 55

3.80   Foods that can make you look younger...56

3.90   Foods and things that can cause body odor 58

3.100   Healthy foods and some risk factors 60

Chapter 4

4.00   Eating habits..62

4.10   Good eating habits 63

4.20   Bad eating habits...64

4.30   Tips to healthy eating..67

4.40   Tips for a healthy looking skin 69

4.50   Steps to changing bad eating habits 71

4.60   How to lose belly fat 73

4.70   The power of what you eat and infections 76

4.80   Other tips to stop you getting sick 78

4.90   Acne pimple and diet 81

Chapter 5

5.00   Nutrients that can make us look a lot younger than our age 82

5.10   Ten tips for an energizing life style 85

5.20   Ten ways to ease your tension 86

5.30   Tips to make you sleep well...88

5.40   Tips to avoid premature aging 90

5.50   Age defying beauty secrets 92

5.60   10 Ways to protect your heart 95

5.70   Factors that cause breast cancer in women...96

5.80   11 Ways to avoid cancer in women 97

5.90   Early signs of breast cancer in women..98

Chapter 6

6.00   Kidney disorder and Prevention 99

6.10   Liver disorders and Prevention..100

6.20   Typhoid fever and Prevention..101

6.30   Arthritis disorder and Prevention 102

6.40   Asthma and Prevention 104

6.50   Tooth disorder and Prevention... 106

6.60   Eye disorders and Prevention 108

6.70   Anemia... 110

6.80   Lung disorder and Prevention 111

6.90   Malaria fever and Prevention... 112

6.100 Acquired immune deficiency syndrome/prevention................... 113

6.110 Gall bladder disorder and Prevention 114

6.120 Thyroid disorder and Prevention 115

Chapter 7

7.00   Infertility in women and men.. 116

7.10   The important qualities of water 122

7.20   Vitamins that give longevity and keep you younger 123

7.30   Preventing hypertension (High Blood Pressure) 129

7.40   Prevention of heart disease (cardiovascular disease)............... 131

7.50   Preventing heart attack... 133

7.60   Preventing stroke.. 136

7.70   Preventing cancer, including prostrate cancer......................... 141

7.80   Stomach ulcer (peptic ulcer) and prevention........................... 144

7.90   Preventing Heart burn 146

7.100 Preventing diabetes.. 149

Chapter 8

8.00   Some medical foods and their healing qualities 151

8.10   Foods with super-healing qualities 151

Conclusion 167

References 169

Index 173

INTRODUCTION

It is quite obvious from research and experience that healthy eating coupled with our life style will be the judging factors as we go through the process of aging. We buy the same foods from the same grocery stores, prepare the same recipes over and over and live within our own family routines with absolute ignorance of certain life styles that may have resulted in the death of some of our older generations. I am sure you already know that if most of your family members suffer from certain ailments and probably die young, it might not just be the heredity factor, but perhaps family cooking and eating routines. However if you are serious about eating healthy, it is necessary that you shake off those generational eating habits and life style. It is also a well known fact that when it comes to eating, some of us tend to have their snacks while working, others are prone to guzzling their beer on an empty stomach, replacing water with beer during their meal, and many other associated eating life style.

Looking young and healthy is an everyday job. Healthy eating coupled with exercise will help you look younger, feel better and live longer. Most of the foods people consume, such as fried chicken, French fries, microwave popcorn, doughnuts, Margarine, cookies, pasties, burgers and many others, contain an artery clogging fat called trans fats, which can cause a lot of disease such as diabetes, high cholesterol, and other health problems to be uncovered later. Many years ago, the resultant affects of most diets was not taken seriously but currently, it has been established that diets that contains large amount of cholesterol and fat, as found in baked ham, margarine butter, French fries, burgers and many others, increase the risk of developing heart disease, diabetes, and other ailments. Many conditions once thought to be the natural progression of aging are now considered to be as a result of poor eating habits and life style. A strong relationship further exist between the level of dietary intake of vitamins and minerals and the development, progression and cure of chronic disorders such as heart, kidney and other related disorders and infections.

Most people think that eating healthy can be tasteless, especially among the younger generation. This notion is further compounded because most of the commercial advertisements promote foods high in calories, fat or sugar and most have not even looked into certain benefits of most fruits, vegetables, whole grains, beans and many others. Many diets out their which have encouraged weight loss and other conditions have worked for most people, however a considerable number seem to abandon such diet half way due to the dissatisfaction of consuming such food on a daily basis, and inevitably going back to their normal tasteful diet. If we want to enjoy a youthful and healthy life style, we must acknowledge that eating healthy improves resistance to colds and infections, reduce the risk of developing acute or chronic diseases, increases resistance to stress and stress related disorders, maintain a feeling of well being, helps in the prevention of premature aging, helps in the maintenance of healthy appearance, improve the outcome of pregnancy and the health of the unborn baby, helps in the regulation of a stable, emotional and social life, and finally, promotes a long and healthy life.

In this research the authors has been able to uncover some of the vital issues relating to healthy eating and life style. They have also tried to look at some of the most common disorders and ways we can prevent the manifestation of such disorders later in life from our eating habits and life style. The research has further looked into other areas which lead to longevity including some healing benefits of certain foods we eat.

While it is important to acknowledge the potential benefits that will prevail based on this research, it is however necessary to consult your physician or seek full professional advice because our body's tends to react differently. An expert or your physician will be in the best position to recommend what is best for you. This study serves as a guide only.

CHAPTER 1

1.00 <u>Good health and good living</u>

Good health and good living is all about watching what you eat and your overall life style. This means the need to watch your calorie intake, fat intake and the need to have regular exercise and to ensure you engage in a reasonable eating pattern. If you keep to these rules, you will obviously look better, feel better and hopefully live longer. Besides, you will always enjoy the compliments from your friends, family, and even strangers who will always wonder what the magic factor is.

Don't be surprise the number of people that will approach you on a weekly or even daily basis to tell them your magic formula. This will not only increase your self esteem, but will encourage you to perfect on your new found image.

I had a grandmother who died at the age of 108 years; she was never hospitalized throughout her life, never used a walking stick, and was relatively active before her death. I suppose she may have even lived longer, if not that her death was accidental through a fall.

I was very close to her and even at a tender age, I was eager to find out why she was the only one still alive amongst all her siblings and friends. I was always carried away, trying to find some facts and knowledge by asking a lot of questions. Based on my findings, I decided to review some of these findings with the present day technology with the help of a specialist company. I have finally come to the conclusion that most of her eating habit and life style are not far from what is expected today, if we anticipate to have a reasonably long life.

The truth is that good health, longevity, and feeling good, is all about healthy eating life style and exercise. We all must be aware of our intake of calories and fat, which will be discussed later in detail. However the truth is that most of us do not know how many calories we consume and the same applies to the type of food and fats we consume. It is always better to monitor our calories intake by writing down everything we eat and drink. The nutritional facts on the food label will help us to come up to our own conclusion on our average calories intake. This also applies to the fats and the type of fats we consume. While the authors will expand on this topic in subsequent headings, it is best to acknowledge that the latest results on how many calories are eaten on average per day are 2,095, with 50% being carbohydrates, 34% being fat, 15% as protein and 2% alcohol. Of course this is only an average figure, because some people will consume a lot more of this average or considerably below. It must be noted that men need more calories to maintain their weight than women.

> **THE TRUTH IS THAT GOOD HEALTH, LONGEVITY AND FEELING GOOD, IS ALL ABOUT HEALTHY EATING, LIFE STYLE AND EXERCISE**

1.10 <u>Common killers of good looks and good health</u>

The aging process is inevitable. While it is obvious that we all want to slow down the speed of the aging process, it is quite obvious that most people actually contribute towards their rate of aging. There are still a considerable number of people who are not willing to accept this reality and quite often they carry on with their normal life style and habits, which will lead to the aging process appearing before their time and resulting in premature aging. Who want to get older and look weaker faster? The obvious answer is that none of us will want to follow this average that will make our face look older faster, which quite often leads towards poor health. We all want that good look and good health which will bring us regular compliments, with high self esteem. If you really want to understand what I am saying try looking at yourself in the mirror and tell me what you see and how you feel. I don't really want to disrespect some fat and unhealthy people out there, but the simple truth is that if you don't like what you see, you will most likely be unhappy and miserable and quite often sensitive to certain comments around you even though they might not really be referring to you. Your self esteem and morale in this instance will not be particularly high. However all is not lost because you can still do something about your situation.

There are certain issues that can result in making us to lose our goods looks and age faster and subsequently leads to poor health.

1. **Life Style**

   Heavy drinkers of alcohol and smokers must be aware that toxins and free radicals contained in them can attack the skin cells, making the skin slower to replace cells that die as a result of these habits. The skin usually dries faster and appears wrinkly and dull.

2. **Lack of exercise and poor diet**

   It is quite obvious that healthy eating along with exercise will make us feel a lot better, improve our looks and subsequently improve our health. We must all try to task our self to achieve this very important area of concern if we want to maintain our looks and good health.

   While we believe that the world is fast changing in the area of beauty, where experts are now able to slow and cope with various symptoms of aging using methods such as the injection procedure, fillers and so on, which serves to reduce wrinkles and the aging lines on the face, however it can be argued that the natural delay is always the best method because there are no guarantees that these conventional methods will always provide the solution to most cases. Another important area that needs to be taken seriously is the area of saturated fat. Diets high in saturated fats increase inflammation, which ages the skin. It also leads to a number of health problems to be uncovered later.

Sweets and refined carbohydrates also raise our blood glucose level, which interferes with the normal repair of collagen and elastic and as a result make us lose those good looks. High intake of these, also lead to a number of health problems.

3. Expression

Are you one of those who tend to come up with facial expressions quite often than normal? While it is difficult to reduce some of these natural habits, it is quite obvious to know that you will not particular look great when compared with some of your friends and families 20 years down the line.

The more expressive a person, it becomes increasingly easy for the skin to thin, waves are seen on the skin more deeply.

Are you one of the moody frowning and angry person who quite often engage your entire face in this angry exercise? If you do that quite often, check yourself out in the next ten years. You will notice that you will most likely be a candidate of a wrinkly forehead. Conversely people who laugh often will most likely have folds of laughter on their cheek as they get older.

4. Certain Habits

Do you always sleep sideways with your cheek stuck to the pillow? This will make you wrinkle fast on that side of the face. If you smoke or drink with a straw you will be most likely making use of more lip muscles and subsequently will register some wrinkles over the years in that area of the face.

Further poor sitting habits such as leaning or bending will indirectly affect the future shape of your body as you get older.

Think about this, are you going to be a hunch back candidate later in life due to this habit.

> **WE ALL WANT THAT GOOD LOOKS AND GOOD HEALTH, WHICH WILL BRING US REGULAR COMPLIMENTS TOGETHER WITH HIGH SELF ESTEEM**

1.20   <u>Its always better to start reasonably early</u>

While the issues of healthy eating and life style can start at any given time irrespective of your age, however we all know that it is always better to start this process reasonably early. No one will want to wait until the manifestation of certain chronic disease or disorder before making that vital decision.

I had a friend years back who is always full of life, he was always cheerful and looked reasonably healthy, however he was a heavy smoker and drinker and rarely cooks in his house. He usually buys most of his foods in the high street and the truth is that he consumes a considerable amount of junk foods. He travels all over the world due to the demands of his job and enjoys a very high income. I was the person closest to him and advised him on a number of occasions to change this life style.

Because he was rarely sick, he uses this as an excuse until one day, the inevitable happened. He felt sick and went for a routine check up and the result was devastating. He had cancer which needed to be treated urgently. This meant he had to undergo an emergency operation, but unfortunately he did not make it. Sad isn't it, only if he had listened. We are all responsible towards the part to our own destruction and doesn't this make us really stupid? I guess most people if given the second chance will turn their life around but unfortunately there will always be the unlucky ones.

Poor nutrition and life style right from our childhood if not addressed as we get older, will result in chronic diseases in adulthood. Eating habit and healthy life style are best developed when we are younger.

> **POOR NUTRITION AND LIFE STYLE RIGHT FROM OUR CHILDHOOD, IF NOT ADDRESSED AS WE GET OLDER WILL RESULT IN CHRONIC DISEASES IN ADULTHOOD.**

1.30 <u>Prevention is always better than cure</u>

I am sure that you will agree with me on this notion. Considering that today a lot of individuals are suffering from different diseases and are spending a consideration amount of money for their treatments which would have been prevented.

It is true that some of these patients lacked the knowledge and given the opportunity they wouldn't have found themselves in their present situation, however a considerable number seem to know that their present situation appears to be an issue of ignorance from their own part.

A couple of years ago, I visited a colleague of mine in the hospital who was suffering from liver disease. He was a heavy alcoholic candidate for a number of years and in his ward, there were other liver disease patients. I got talking to a number of them because I needed to find out why they indulged in a habit they knew quite obviously will eventually kill them.

Surprisingly, a considerable number where unaware of the dangers and acknowledged the fact that if they know what they know now, they will not go to the extreme that kept them in their present situation.

A considerable number also acknowledged the fact that they knew the consequences but thought it will never happen to them, while a few proportion acknowledged the dangers and put their situation down to depression.

The truth is that none of them wanted to die and while some needed that initial education on the dangers which would have prevented their situation, others would have benefited from counseling and other necessary professional help. Most of the patients appear to be malnourished and paid little attention to what they eat. In fact a number of them were drinking alcohol on an empty stomach, with absolute disregard about their health.

They appeared to be on a very poor diet, which further compounded their situation. Lack of balanced diet, provides avenue for diseases, while a balanced diet provides the preventative measures for diseases.

Having all the nutrients such as carbohydrates, fats, proteins, vitamins and minerals, in the right proportion, can save us from a lot of diseases.

According to medical experts and research, stress can also lead to a number of diseases in our body. This is because stress affects the functioning of the heart, which plays the role of pumping blood to all parts of our body.

On this note, stress prevention and management is very important to keep us away from the doctors.

Exercising regularly is another route for the prevention of disease. This is because when we exercise it enhance the functioning of various part of the body and subsequently prepare our body ready enough to fight off diseases.

If we adhere to all there rules, we will be preventing most of these diseases rather than treating them.

**A LOT OF INDIVIDUALS ARE SUFFERING
FROM DIFFERENT DISEASES AND ARE SPENDING
A CONSIDERABLE AMOUNT OF MONEY FOR THERE
TREATMENT,
WHICH WOULD HAVE BEEN PREVENTED**

1.40   Its never too late to say yes to change

Yes, perhaps you are thinking about your age, and have given up already to a change of diet, healthy eating and life style; however the reality is that it is never too late to turn things around, and add a few more years to your life span, and better quality of life.

No matter your age, the value of exercise and nutrition is not questionable. No matter your age, everything you do in life, I don't care whether good or bad, don't blame God, don't even blame the devil, don't blame your parents or even me, blame yourself, because you are in control of your destiny. The thoughts you think, the words you say, the foods you eat on a daily basis, and your exercise routine, all accounts for your own good or bad.

I know we will all become old one day, but doesn't it really make sense to think towards looking strong and healthy and being able to do those things we like doing during our senior years. Our body is like our favorite car.

I remember when I first bought a car, I really took care of this car to ensure that it drives me around were ever I want to go, I kept the car in a very good condition and serviced the car regularly. But quite often we tend to look after those things that we admire and forget the most important one, that is our self. It is quite obvious that no matter how well maintained your car, if you are not healthy, you will struggle to drive the car around.

The more things you do to help your healthy, the more you will be able to get out of your body. If you ignore this fact, then you will be obviously a candidate of several diseases as you get older. You will get sick and tired, you will obviously visit your doctor or end up in hospital, and if you are likely to come out of the hospital, you may decide to go on holidays with the notion that it will help you get better, but the truth is that the problem will always be there.

Therefore we must first start early or reasonably early and stop the problems and diseases on their tracks. There are a lot of people out there who eat a reasonable balanced diet, but don't exercise and conversely there are others who exercise and eat a lot of junk foods and the reality is that we must make the bold decision to deprive ourselves some of these tasty meals we enjoy and eat some few things that appear to be tasteless in order to achieve our goal. This also applies to exercise, which will subsequently give us some certain discomfort which we tend to dislike, but helps our body.

A lot of older people tend to sit around all day long, their muscles become weaker, and they lose their strength and energy over time and I know you don't want to be one of those statistics. Besides the balanced diet, exercising is like a catalyst, which will kick start, our body system, our defense mechanism to diseases, our digestion, our waste elimination, our sex life and hence everything about us depends on circulation which is aided by our exercise.

If for instance you are around 70 years old and have never exercised, and you decide to exercise for 6-8 weeks, you will most likely double your strength and endurance.

Studies have even proved that people in their 90's who were all put on a weight training programme doubled their strength and endurance. The truth in that no matter your age, you can always make that bold decision for a healthy and enjoyable life style.

**THE MORE THINGS YOU DO TO
HELP YOUR HEALTH; THE MORE
YOU WILL BE ABLE TO GET
OUT OF YOUR BODY**

1.50 <u>You are what you eat</u>

I don't really want to sound offensive or rude but take a good look at yourself in the mirror first and foremost do you like what you see or could you have looked better. Secondly, think about what you usually eat and drink and finally blame yourself for the outcome if you don't like what you see.

The reality is that if you live on junk and fast foods, you will probably be fat, unhealthy and weak when compared with the person that tend to embark on balanced diet, exercise regularly, the obvious outcome will be fit and healthy looking.

Most of us seem to be ignorant of what we eat and we must begin to acknowledge our shortcomings towards the way we feel and look as a result of our eating habits and life style. We often tend to find it difficult to break away from our favorite tasty meals and drink and it usually requires a bombshell like a health scare from our doctor before we start making the necessary sacrifice. We shouldn't wait until we are pushed to the wall before disciplining ourselves for our own health benefits.

We must seek healthier foods that are overall low in sodium or saturated fats and higher in fiber. This will be looked at more in detail in subsequent chapters.

If for instance one or two people in your family have type 2 diabetes or heart disease, it means that there are perhaps others around the dinner table who could be at risk as well.

Ignorance is a big killer, and in circumstances like this, the applicable families must try to do something about this or risk registering further chronic disorders in the family. We all know the stress and monetary consequences of this ignorance, which should have been prevented.

WE OFTEN TEND TO FIND IT DIFFICULT TO BREAK AWAY FROM OUR FAVORITE TASTY MEALS AND DRINK AND IT USUALLY REQUIRE A BOMBSHELL LIKE A HEALTH SCARE FROM OUR DOCTOR BEFORE MAKING THE NECESSARY SACRIFICES

1.60   Healthy life style that can lead to longevity

Longevity certainly is something every one desires of, but attaining that magic age certainty doesn't come that cheap and we all have to work towards it. Experts agree that the key to longevity goes along with healthy eating, regular exercise, and a healthy life style. We must also be aware of our family history of diseases and make a considerable effort to avoid being part of that statistics.

With so much information available concerning a well balanced diet, it will only take absolute ignorance not to catch our attention.

Studies have shown that diet that contain large amount of cholesterol and fat, increases our risk of developing heart disease, cancer, hypertension and other related disorders. Of course fat is an essential nutrient everyone needs to stay alive and healthy and is a valuable energy source and carries fat soluble vitamins needed for proper growth and development. However, too much of this fat especially saturated fat, to be discussed later in detail is not good for our health.

We must also ensure that we exercise regularly and cut down on certain habits such as alcohol consumption, smoking, other obvious bad habits and most importantly eating a well balanced diet to be discussed later, usually propels us towards longevity.

First you must eat a variety of nutrient rich foods. We need more than 40 different nutrients for good health and no single food supplies the relevant nutrients. Your daily food selection should include things like, bread and other wholegrain products, fruits and vegetables, dairy product, meat, fish and other protein foods. Your consumption will depend on your calorie need. Usually the nutritional facts in food labels will usually prove handy. Studies for instance have shown that most people do not eat much of whole grains, fruits and vegetables.

We must also maintain a healthy weight through a combination of our diet and exercise. You ideal weight is largely dependent on your sex, height, age and heredity. Excess body fat, will obviously increase your chances of suffering from heart disease, diabetes, high blood pressure, stroke, cancer and other related disorders and being too thin also have its own drawbacks, such as the risk of suffering from menstrual irregularities, osteoporosis, and other related disorders.

We must eat moderately and select our portion to be of a reasonable size. A number of food guide pyramids will usually give an indication of what is moderate and too much.

We must eat regular meals, and shouldn't skip meals. Skipping meals usually leads to out of control hunger which subsequently leads us to overeating. A lot of people tend to snack between meals but be watchful that the snacking does not end up becoming the entire meal.

You must reduce but try not to eliminate certain meals. If your favorite meals appear to be high in fat, salt or sugar, the main concern is to reduce much of this food you eat and how often you eat them.

You must balance your choice of food over time. When consuming some foods that are high in fat, salt or sugar you can select other foods that are low in these ingredients.

If you are out on any food group one day, make up for it the next day. Your choice of food over several days should fit together into a healthy pattern.

You must try to observe your diet pitfalls. Observe your body chemistry each time you eat a certain food and how you feel for the rest of the day, then reduce the intake of such food or seek professional solution. The idea in not to eliminate those vital nutrients entirely but to reduce on their intake or look for a substitute that accepts your body chemistry.

Make changes to your diet gradually if you have taken that bold decision. Take it one step at a time to remedy excesses and deficiencies with modest changes that can add up to a positive acceptable eating habit.

Finally there are certain foods that have proved to increase our life span.

1. **Broccoli**
   According to studies from experts, broccoli contains more vitamins C than oranges, more calcium than a glass of milk, as well as natural fibers more than a lot of bread wheat. It also contains antioxidants. Broccoli is also one of the many vegetables that contain anti-carcinogens that can stimulate the body against cancer causing substances. It also prevents cataracts, heart disease, arthritis, ulcers and many other diseases.

2. Chamomile

Chamomile flowers are used to relax the nerves, reduce stress and pressure. The less stressed you are, the lower the chances of developing a variety of diseases caused by stress. Chamomile also helps to detoxify the body by removing toxic materials through the kidney. Chamomile can be consumed as dried food or brewed. It can also be dipped into hot water like tea.

3. Cranberries

Cranberries contains vitamin C, chemically it eradicates bacterial substances. This fruit helps to protect the entry of harmful bacteria into the organs of our body.

4. Fish oil

Some fish such as salmon, macharel, or anchory is known for producing omega 3, which can lower cholesterol levels, as well as protecting us from strokes, and blood clots in the brain.

5. Lemon

Lemon is a close relative of citrus fruits that contain lot of vitamin C. Addition of lemon in our diet maintains the beauty of the face. Lemon juice anti-bacterial properties help us to fight off infections such as thrush in the mouth, and sore throat.

YOU MUST TRY TO OBSERVE
YOU DIET PITFALLS

1.70 Foods that burn fats

While exercise is a fantastic way of burning fat and keep us looking healthy and sexy, there are also foods that burn fat by increasing our metabolism. Some studies have proven that some foods do in fact increase the rate at which our body burns calories.

For example, there is a slight thermogenic effect from capsaicin in hot pepper. Well controlled studies has also proven that a compound in green tea called epigallo-catechin gallate (EGCG), give a small but significant increase in 24 hour metabolic rate. It usually takes 3-4 cups of green tea to get the necessary amount 270-300mg of EGCG, or it can also be obtained from green tea extract supplements.

Also a study published in the European journal of clinical nutrition, found that a dose of hot pepper only increase metabolism by 21 calories, green tea extract fared a little better. Research from Switzerland found an average 24 hours increase in metabolism of 79 calories.

The truth is that green tea is extremely healthy, and it is a good recommendation in a beverage, however what will help you burn fat more is a diet consisting of nutrient dense natural foods and putting together your meals to maximize satiety and also choosing some of the foods that have a lower caloric density and a higher thermic effect of digestion.

Dietary Thermogenesis and the thermic effect of food

All foods are thermogemic because the body must use energy to digest them. This is known as the "thermic effect of food" (TEF) or "specific dynamic action of food".

However, not all foods have the same thermic effect. Dietary fat has the lowest thermic effect and the most thermogenic food is lean protein from solid foods especially the following.

a. Chicken breast
b. Turkey breast
c. Game meats (venison elk etc)
d. Bison buffalo
e. Very lean red meat such as top round and lean sarlon

f. Almost all types of fish
g. Egg whites

Studies has proven that the thermic effect of protein is the highest of all the macronutrients, requiring about 30% of the calories it contains just for digestion and processing. Further lean protein foods suppress our appetite.

This is one of the reasons that a fat loss diet calls for a lean protein food at every meal. It is also no coincidence that body builders, are the leanest muscular athletes around the world.

When you combine thermogenic lean protein foods, with the right amounts and types of essential fats, add in plenty of green vegetables and just the right amount of natural starchy carbohydrates, your body will turn into a turbo-charged fat burning machine.

Here are some simple 3 steps formulas to put together a fat burning meal.

1. Select a green vegetable or fibrous vegetable such as asparagus, green beans, broccoli, brussel sprouts, cauliflower, salad vegetables etc.
2. Combine these with one of the lean protein, previously mentioned above.
3. The lean protein and fibrous carb forms the foundation of your fat burning meal, from here add natural starchy carbs or grains such as brown rice, oats or sweet potatoes, in the amount your calorie needs require and to the degree your body can tolerate them, fruits are also good but focus even more on the green and fibrous vegetables and then see the result.

There are known foods that increase the rate at which our body burns fat but not in the magnitude detailed above, these foods are:

1. Cayenne pepper
2. Ginger
3. Cinnamon
4. Apples and berries
5. Citrus fruits
6. Soy beans
7. Essential fatty acids (EFAs)
8. Garlic
9. Sea weed
10. Green tea

Eating these foods will not work on their own you must always maintain a healthy diet and exercise routine.

> **ALL FOODS ARE THERMOGENIC BECAUSE THE BODY MUST USE ENERGY TO DIGEST THEM**

CHAPTER 2

2.00 Diets

We all know that certain group of people and countries tend to live longer and appear stronger with relatively low disease rate. The obvious truth is that all people blessed with longevity tend to eat a diet based on whole grain, beans, vegetables, local fruits and very small portion of meat or dairy products. They also tend to eat very low-calorie meats, with a very small amount of fat intake in the range of 15%.

We must all pay attention to what we are eating and drinking, this will help us know how we can improve our diet. It wouldn't be a bad idea to keep food diaries for our personal reference.

Don't expect too much from yourself very fast, chances is that it will take in the region of one to two months before the routine becomes reality and hence form part of your life style.

Most people are usually skeptical at first about changing their diets, having gotten use to those tasty foods they are very much use to, but will it require a health scare from your doctor to force you to make this important decision of change?

> **WE MUST ALL PAY ATTENTION
> ON WHAT WE ARE EATING
> AND DRINKING, THIS WILL HELP US
> KNOW HOW WE CAN IMROVE OUR DIET**

2.10 Choosing your daily diet

Choosing your daily diet should follow the four food group outlined below;

1. It is very necessary that you limit the fat on your diet to not more than 30% of your total calories and cholesterol to 300mg/day or less.

2. Increase the fiber in your diet, limit processed refined or commercial convenience foods that are often high in fat, sugar, salt, cholesterol or highly processed ingredient.

3. Choose a variety of wholegrain nutrients foods every day.

4. You must be moderate in your food selection and portion size. While taking note of the recommended calorie intake applicable to you. Men need 2000-2500 calories to maintain their weight and need 1600-2000 calories to lose weight, while women need 1,600 to 2,000 calorie to maintain weight and 1,200 to 1,600 calories to lose weight.

> **MEN NEED 2000-2500 CALORIES TO MAINTAIN**
> **WEIGHT AND 1600-2000 CALORIES TO LOSE WEIGHT**
> **WHILE WOMEN NEED 1600-2000 CALORIES TO MAINTAIN**
> **WEIGHT AND 1,200-1600 CALORIES TO LOSE WEIGHT**

2.20   **Balanced diet**

A balanced diet is one that has all the vitamins, minerals and other nutrients optimal amount. Eating a balanced diet means choosing a wide variety of foods and drinks from all food groups. It will further require eating certain things in moderation, which contains saturated fats Trans fat, cholesterol, refined sugar, salt, alcohol etc. The purpose is to consume nutrients you require for your health at the recommended levels. To achieve a balanced diet, it will require eating fruits, vegetables, whole grains, low or no fat dairy products, fish, lean animal proteins. Fish is recommended at least two times a week, beans, nuts and seeds are advisable and unsaturated fats seem to be the best, such as olive oil.

Your balanced diet must be designed at your own calorie level and portion size. The idea is to get the most nutrients for the calories by choosing foods with a high nutrient density. Nutrients dense foods provide a considerable amount of vitamins and minerals, with relatively less calories, such as fresh fruits and vegetables, lean meat, fish, whole grains and beans. Low nutrients dense foods have lots of calories and little vitamins such as candy bars, soda, doughnuts etc.

The key to achieving balanced diet depends of on you, you need to establish your goal and decide on which food groups you will like to eat, and then figure out which food groups that appear to be missing. You must address issues such as eating too much fats, sugar, salt, fried foods etc. The bottom line is,

1. To eat the right amount of foods based on how active you will be.
2. To eat a variety of foods from the recommended foods groups.

The range of food in your diet should include

a. Plenty of fruits and vegetables.
b. Bread, rice, potatoes, pasta and other starchy foods and choosing wholegrain varieties.
c. Some milk and dairy foods.
d. Some meat, fish, eggs, beans and other non-dairy sources of protein.
e. Small amount of foods high in fat and sugar.

Eating well is the key to maintaining good health which can lead to longevity. Some important healthy eating tips include;

a. Base your meal on starchy foods which gives you energy, and tailor this based on how active you will be.

b. Eat lots of fruits and vegetables daily. Eat at least five portions of a variety of fruits and vegetables daily.

c. Eat at least two portions of fish every week, including one portion of oily fish such as sardine or mackerel.

d. Cut down on saturated fats and sugar

e. Eat less salt no more than 6g a day

f. Exercise regularly and keep a healthy weight

g. Drink plenty of water, at least 6-8 glass or other fluids daily.

h. Do not skip breakfast, because it gives you the initial energy you need for the day.

YOUR BALANCE DIET MUST BE DESIGNED AT YOUR OWN CALORIE LEVEL AND PORTION SIZE IS PARAMOUNT

2.30 **Designing a balanced diet**

Designing a balanced diet revolves around the recommended food groups. Some of these food groups are;

1. The fruit and vegetable group, these are foods which are reliable sources of fiber, vitamin C, vitamin A and folic acid. Some of these fruits are apples, oranges, carrots, tomatoes, lettuce, cabbage, green, pumpkin etc.
2. The whole grain and cereal group, they are usually high in vitamin B, iron, other minerals, and fiber. Examples are Oat meal, brown rice, whole wheat, noodles, wheat berries, barley or millet etc.
3. The low fat milk group, they are good sources of calcium, protein, vitamin B2 etc. Examples are non-fat or low fat milk, non fat or low fat yoghurt, low fat cheese or low fat cottage cheese etc.
4. The lean meat legume group. They are good sources of iron, protein, zinc, vitamin B, and phosphorus etc. Examples are lean meat, chicken or fish, kidney beans, black beans, soy bean, peanut and egg etc.

Follow these four group plan with regular exercise and you will enjoy a healthy life and reduce the risk of developing cardiovascular diseases, cancer, obesity and other related disorders. It must be noted that a diet high in fat such as saturated fat, (vegetable oil, palm oil, beef, butter, all fatty foods), is associated with an increased risk for developing heart (cardiovascular) disease, hypertension, stroke, cancer, and other disorders. Triglycendes are the fats found in vegetable oils, beefs, butter and all fatty foods. Triyglycendes are also found in the blood and are the storage form of fat in the body.

Dietary fats come in a variety of forms including visible fats, such as butter, sour cream, cream cheese, margarine, vegetable shortening, vegetable oils and the visible fat surrounding meat or in chicken skin. These fats must be consumed in a small quantity.

A high fiber diet is associated with a reduced risk for colon cancer, cardiovascular disease, diabetes, hypertension, stroke, and other disorders. Example of high fiber foods are bran in whole wheat and oats, pectin in apples, locust bean gum, fiber in whole grain bread, cereals, vegetables, fruits, cooked dried beans, peas, and insoluble fibers such as wheat bran are associated with a reduced risk of colon cancer and intestinal diseases, while soluble fibers such as pectin in apples and oats bran, reduce blood cholesterol and sugar levels and subsequently the risk of diabetes and cardiovascular disease. Low fat nutritional foods include;

1. Non fat milk or yogurt
2. Low fat milk or yogurt
3. Egg-only the white
4. Whole wheat bread
5. Oat bran (hot cereal)
6. Puffed wheat, rice, millet or corn, grape, nuts, wheat, barley, and corn cereal
7. Bran, brown rice, millet, whole wheat flour grains
8. Fruits (fresh), fresh vegetables
9. Tomatoes products
10. Pumpkin, banboo shoot
11. Soy bean, kidney beans, all beans
12. Apple, grape fruit, orange, pineapple
13. Plantain, bananas, potatoes etc.

Key to designing a healthy diet for one day

A healthy diet includes a combination of foods and nutrients from the recommended groups and supports our body physically and emotionally. Certain foods such as saturated fats should be minimized or avoided including sugars. While healthy foods such as fruits, vegetables, should be encouraged.

In designing a healthy diet take the following steps

1. Start with a healthy balanced breakfast, which will provide the initial needed energy for instance, one piece or half cup of fresh fruit, whole grain food, such as oats meal, or one cup of whole grain cereal, a reasonable portion of lean protein such as I cup of low fat milk, and some healthy fat such as one tea spoon of milk. If you don't consume fat at breakfast, then use Omega 3 fatty acid supplements.

2. Go for a mid day meal three to five hours after your breakfast. If your lunch occurs more than five hours later a mid-morning snack such as fruit and yogurt is advisable. Fill half your lunch plate with vegetables such as leafy green. Studies have proved that four or more servings, of vegetables per day, leads to improved heart health and longevity (Mayo clinic). Fill one quarter of your plate with complex carbohydrates such as 2/3 cup brown rice or one plain baked potato. The remaining quarter should contain lean protein 1/3 oz chicken grilled, 3 ounces of fish or ½ to 1 cup of beans. Add some healthy fat such as 1 to 2

tea spoon of olive oil to your meal as salad dressing or to add flavor to rice or poultry.

3. Have a mid-afternoon snack three to four hours after your lunch. Your snack must contain more than one food group, with some important nutrients. Snacks with some protein and carbohydrates are good choice, because they will help support you blood sugar levels. (American diabetes Association). A cut of low fat cottage cheese topped with berries, one slice whole grain toast, topped with I tea spoon peanut butter and 3 ounces turkey, sliced served on whole grain crackers is a good option.

4. Have a balanced dinner meal at least two hours before your bed time. If the meal is consumed too close to bed time when the body is winding down, sleep can be disturbed. Choose at least two servings' of vegetables such as salad steamed or grilled veggies, a healthy carbohydrate such as one cup of whole grain pasta topped with tomato sauce and lean protein such as 3 ounces of fish, poultry, beans or tofu. If you desire dessert, make a choice low in sugar, such as fresh fruit, topped with non fat yogurt.

5. Drink at least 6-8 cups of water throughout the day and minimize or avoid alcohol and sugary beverages such as soda. Herbal teas, fresh fruits or vegetable juices are acceptable.

> ## A HEALTHY DIET INCLUDES A VARIETY OF FOODS AND NUTRIENTS FROM THE RECOMMENDED GROUPS

2.40 Calories

A calorie is a measurement of energy in food. Thus a calorie is a unit of energy. When we say that something contains 150 calories, this relates to how much energy your body could get from eating or drinking it.

Our bodies need calories for energy and eating too much calories will require burning them off through exercise or other activities, to prevent us from gaining weight.

Most foods we buy in the supermarket or groceries will normally have a label to give us an idea of their calorie contents which will help us control our calorie consumption.

The problem with calorie intake is that most people appear to be ignorant about how many calories they are consuming, however the best approach is to write down everything you eat or drink. You can use the nutritional facts on food labels as a guide.

The latest results of how many calories are eaten; on average per day is 2095, with 50% being carbohydrates, 34% being fat, 15% protein and 2% alcohol.

On average men need 2000 to 2500 calories per day to maintain their weight and 1,600 to 2,000 calories per day to lose weight. Women on average need 1,600-2000 calories per day to maintain their weight, and 1,200-1600 calories to lose weight.

A calorie counter usually measures the rate you are burning off those calories during exercise. Exercise is very important in burning calories. Without proper exercise our body will not burn off the calories and fat that it needs to. Usually a lot of people tend to worry about the right time to eat in a situation of exercise. It is best to eat more than two hours but less than four hours before exercising. High fat or sugar meals are not recommended before exercising, but it is necessary that we drink some water before exercising.

Your weight is the factor in determining how many calories are burned. Calorie counters use your weight combined with the intensity of activity to find out how many calories we burned. Some activities usually burn off more calories than others. On average the following calories are burned within an hour depending on the activities. For instance walking = 238 calories, basket ball =545 calories, bicycling=

545 calories, in line skating =477 calories, running 5mph= 545 calories, bowling= 204 calories, golf= 306 calories, dancing= 306 calories, ice hockey= 545 calories, skiing= 477 calories, tennis= 477 calories, weight lifting= 204 calories, swimming= 545 calories, stretching= 272 calories, jogging= 477 calories.

For people trying to reduce calories intake, they must reduce the amount of sugar and cooking oil used. Steam or gill all meat instead of frying, select fiber rich foods, always read a food label and consult a dietician.

On average most foods have their calorie contents written on the package, but we must watch out for the serving size to ensure we are abreast with our calorie intake. Fruits and vegetables are usually low in calorie, skim milk reduces calories and fish and chicken without the skin are preferable to red meat, to reduce calories.

There are some vegetables and fruits that are classed as negative calories (burn off calories). The usual ones are cauliflower, celery, lettuce, broccoli, cucumbers, grapefruits, peaches, strawberries, and melon etc.

Some of us think that we have to burn off all the calories we eat or else we will gain weight. This is not true because our body need some calories in order to operate. For instance to keep our heart beats and our lung to breath.

Calorie in children is also an interesting topic. Children are all different in sizes and each person body burns calories at different rates. Therefore there isn't one perfect number of calories that a kid should eat, but there is a recommended range for most school age kids in the region of 1,600-2500 calories per day. It must be noted that people who are more active will need more calorie intake, than their less active counterparts.

> **THE PROBLEM WITH CALORIE INTAKE IS THAT MOST PEOPLE APPEAR TO BE IGNORANT ABOUT HOW MANY CALORIES THEY ARE CONSUMING**

2.50 Calorie dense food

Calorie dense foods are those that have large amount of calories for their portion size. Calorie dense foods tend to be high in fat and/or sugar. Usually all proteins and all carbohydrates contain four calories per gram, while all fats contain nine calories per gram and some foods are more. For those trying to gain weight this type of food will be helpful.

Typical calorie dense foods include fatty meats, salami, candy bars, rice crackers, cookies, potato chips, anything which is fried, cola, beer, except low calorie ones, ice cream etc.

These foods tend to be high in sugar and /or fat.

When we try to make necessary adjustments to our weight gain diet to include more calories, we must do so in a healthy manner. We do not just look at consuming calories, but must also look at the nutritional value of foods, for instance fruits and vegetables which has very good nutritional values.

Fibrous carbohydrates and vegetables such as lettuce, asparagus, cucumber, broccoli, are also known to be very low in calories and because of their high fiber contents, our body tend to have a difficult time in trying to absorb the calorie contents.

For people who want to gain weight, minimize the consumption of vegetable and replace them with simple carbohydrates such as fruits with a higher calorie density. This is because simple carbohydrates are more concentrated and they contain less fiber. Fruit juice is even more concentrated than eating the fruit itself. Fruits and fruit juices appear to contribute considerably to any weight gain programmed.

Complex carbohydrates (starches) such as whole grains, pasta, cereals, potatoes and rice also have higher calorie densities than fibrous carbohydrates. A typical serving of pasta contains about 800-1000 calories. Complex carbohydrates are good food for gaining weight.

Now looking at the issue of fat, there is a common misunderstanding that all fats are bad for us. This is not true because there are good and bad fats to be discussed in detail later. It must be noted that a diet high in fat such as saturated fat (vegetable oil, palm oil, margarine and all fatty foods) is associated with an increase risk for developing heart (cardiovascular) disease, hypertension, stroke, cancer and other disorders.

Fats have a major part to playing in the calorie content of foods; therefore they are part of the consideration. We must note that fat should be in the range of 15-25% of our total calories intake; however most of our calories should be coming from carbohydrates and protein. In small amounts, unsaturated healthy fats are not only good for us, but can help us gain weight more quickly. Just one table spoon of flaxseed oil and two table spoon of peanut butter would add some reasonable calories to our daily diet.

In addition a healthy diet can be supplemented by protein supplements. It is often difficult to eat enough protein each day from normal foods. Therefore it is necessary to supplement if necessary. We must ensure that the weight gain supplement is a good mix of both protein and carbohydrates and doesn't contain a lot of sugar. For instance a post workout shake containing 40 grams of protein, 80 grams of carbohydrates and 2 grams of fat will provide almost 500 calories.

Therefore in summary, for adding more calories to your diet, continue eating the same healthy foods, just eat more of them. Replace low calorie foods, with high calorie foods. Eating salad all day will not do you any good if you want to gain weight. Focus on eating plenty of starchy carbohydrates, including whole grains, pastas, rice, and potatoes. Ensure that your fat intake is not more than 15-25% of your total calories. Some added good fats will help you to grain weight.

But a word of advice, your need to eat more calories doesn't give you the avenue to engulf yourself with unnecessary unhealthy foods. You must ensure a healthy choice of food.

**CALORIE DENSE FOODS TEND
TO BE HIGH IN FAT AND/OR SUGAR**

2.60 **Nutrients and Essential nutrients**

A nutrient is a substance obtained from the diet and used in the body to promote the growth, maintenance, and repair of our tissue. The bottom line is that

1. Nutrients are essential for cell growth, maintenance and repair.
2. Nutrients provide energy to enable our body to function efficiently.
3. Nutrient along with fiber and water are essential to our good health. While we acknowledge that nutrients can work alone, each depends upon the others to provide the best results. The main nutrients are the macronutrients and micronutrients.

Macronutrients

Macronutrients are necessary for our good health; they play a part in breaking down carbohydrates and fats which provide energy to the body. They also assist in the absorption of protein which provides the building blocks necessary for cell growth and repair.

Micronutrients

Vitamins and minerals do not in themselves provide energy but micronutrients depend on them to regulate the release of energy from food.

1. Vitamins are organic substances
2. They activate enzymes, which are proteins that act as catalysts to speed up biological reactions that take place in our body.
3. Our body produces a certain amount of vitamin D and K but all other vitamins come from our diet or supplements.

Minerals are inorganic substances that originate from rocks, and Ores and enter the food chain through the soil.

1. We get minerals either by eating plants grown on mineral rich soil or by eating animals that has fed on these plants.
2. Calcium, magnesium, and phosphorous are the major constituents of bone.
3. Sodium and potassium controls our body's water balance.
4. Other minerals—chromium, iron, and magnesium are needed for various chemical processes that take place in the body
5. Omega fatty acids and

6. Phytonutients also referred to as phytochemicals are compounds that act as a natural defense system in plants and also have a beneficial effect in our health.

Essential Nutrients

An essential nutrient is one that cannot be produced by the body at all or in adequate amount for maintaining good health and must be obtained from diet or food. Some lists of essential nutrients includes, vitamins, dietary minerals, essential fatty acids, and essential amino acids. Human beings require for instance external sources of ascorbic acid, known as vitamin C in their nutrition.

Mainly essential nutrients are toxic in large doses; some can be taken in amounts larger than required in a typical diet with no apparent side effect.

> **NUTRIENTS ARE ESSENTIAL FOR CELL GROWTH, MAINTAINANCE AND REPAIR**

2.70 **Nutrients dense foods**

Nutrients dense foods are foods that provides large amount of vitamins and minerals, with a small amount of calories. Example are fruits and vegetables, whole grain bread and cereals, cooked dried beans, peas, low fat and non fat dairy products, fish, chicken without the skin, lean meat, oats meals etc.

Nutrients dense foods are reach in nutrients when compared with their calories contents.

Foods are known to fulfill three basic needs.

1. To provide energy
2. Support new tissue growth and repair
3. To help regulate metabolism.

And these requirements are the characteristics of nutrients which consist of carbohydrates, fat, protein, vitamins, minerals and water. Foods such as whole grain breads, cereals, rice, beans, pastas, vegetables and fruits are nutrients dense foods because they are not only high in carbohydrates, but also supply others nutrients, such as vitamins, minerals, protein, and fiber. The key point to note in this instance is that the vitamins and minerals content must be considerably higher than the calorie content. By comparison, sweet foods that are considerably high in sugar, such as candy bars, doughnuts, cookies etc, contain carbohydrates but they are not considered nutrients dense because they are obviously high in fat contents with a considerable low vitamins and minerals contents.

Nutrients dense Carbohydrates appear to have considerable acceptance over fats and sugary foods because they have fewer calories for a given amount than foods with a high fat or sugary content.

Essential nutrients during pregnancy

A low fat, high fiber, nutrients dense diet comprising of all vitamins and minerals, especially vitamin A, C, E, D, and B plus vitamins such as calcium and iron etc.

The following diets must be observed during pregnancy

1. Eat at least two servings of milk product or take calcium daily.
2. Eat considerable fruits and vegetables daily

3. Eat four servings of energy foods daily such as whole grains products, cooked and dried beans, the good sources of carbohydrates and proteins.

4. Eat good servings of organ meat such as liver, heart of beef, lean meats, fish and chicken without the skin.

5. Doctors usually advice on 30-60 milligram of iron daily because it is almost impossible to get this much iron from diet.

6. Avoid excess Sugar and salt.

7. Drink at least eight glasses of water daily.

8. Avoid hot spicy meals and caffeinated products.

> **NUTRIENTS DENSE FOODS ARE REACH IN NUTRIENTS WHEN NOT WATER COMPARED WITH THEIR CALORIES CONTENS**

2.80 Antioxidants

Antioxidants are substances produced in the body or nutrients supplied in the diet that neutralizes harmful substances called free radicals that are associated with diseases such as cardiovascular disease, cancer, premature aging etc.

The bottom line is that antioxidants protect our cell against the effects of free radicals. Free radicals are molecules produced when our body breaks down food or by environmental exposures like tobacco smoke, radiation, etc. Free radicals can damage cells and usually contributes to heart diseases, cancer and other disorders.

Antioxidants substances include

1. Beta-carotene
2. Lutein
3. Lycopene
4. Selenium
5. Vitamin A
6. Vitamin C
7. Vitamin E

Antioxidants are found in many foods such as vegetable oils, seeds, wheat, germ and nuts, organ meats, sea foods, fish, lean meat, whole grain, brown rice, oat meals, whole wheat, dark yellow vegetables, fruits, dark green, which are good sources of vitamin E and subsequently orange juice, strawberries, tomato juice, cabbage, potato, green peas, pineapple, corn on the hob, which are good sources of vitamin C.

An overview of foods rich in antioxidants are

1. Beta-carotene is found in many foods that are orange in color, including sweet potatoes, carrots, cantaloupe, squash, apricots, pumpkin and mangoes. Some green leafy vegetables including collard greens, spinach, and kale are quite rich in beta-carotene.
2. Lutein is popular for its added benefits for healthy eyes and can be obtained by eating green leafy vegetables such as collard greens, spinach and kale.
3. Lycopene can be found in tomatoes, water melon, guava, papaya, apricots, pink grape fruit and blood oranges. From estimates, 85% of American dietary intake of lycopene comes from tomatoes and tomato products.

4. Selenium is a component of antioxidant enzymes, foods such as rice, and wheat are the main sources of selenium in some countries. However in America, meats and bread are the major sources of selenium.

5. Vitamin A is another form of antioxidant substance and foods rich in vitamin A includes livers, sweet potatoes, carrots, milk, egg yolks, mozzarella, cheese etc.

6. Vitamin C is another form of antioxidant substance and can be found in foods such as fish, poultry, beef, cereals, fruits and vegetables etc.

7. Vitamin E follows suit as an antioxidant substance and can be found in many oils, including wheat germ, safflower, corn, soybean oils, mangoes, nuts, broccoli etc.

**ANTIOXIDANTS PROTECT OUR CELLS
AGAINST THE EFFECTS OF FREE
RADICALS**

2.90 Enzymes

An Enzyme is a compound that acts as a catalyst in starting a chemical reaction. They are the products of amino acid in the body. At any given time all the work being done inside any cell is being done by enzymes.

The purpose of an enzyme in a cell is to allow the cell to carry out chemical reactions very quickly. These reactions allow the cell to build things or take things apart as needed and this is how a cell grows and reproduces.

Enzymes are made from amino acids, and they are proteins. When an enzyme is formed, it is made by stringing together 100 to 1000 amino acids in a unique order. The chain of amino acids then folds into a specific shape. The shape allows the enzymes to carry out specific chemical reactions. An enzyme acts as a very efficient catalyst for specific chemical reactions. The enzymes speeds that reaction up considerably. For instance, the sugar maltose is made from two glucose molecules bonded together. The enzyme maltase is shaped in such a way that it can break the bond and free the two glucose pieces. The only thing maltase can do is to break maltose molecules and it can do this very rapidly and effectively. Subsequently other types of enzymes can put atoms and molecules together. Therefore breaking molecules apart and putting molecules together is what enzymes do, and there is a specific enzyme for each chemical reaction needed to make the cell work effectively.

We have all had about people who are lactose intolerant or perhaps you may be suffering from this problem without knowing.

The problem here arises because the sugar in milk-lactose does not get broken into glucose components and as a result of this, it cannot be digested. Hence the intestinal cells of lactase intolerant people do not produce lactase which is the enzyme needed to break down lactose and this subsequently leads to digestive problems. A person who is lactose intolerant can swallow a drop of lactase before drinking milk and this problem will be solved.

There are three major different types of enzymes at work within our body and within these three types are nearly 3,000 different kinds of enzymes. Each kind has certain specific tasks to carry out and we need most of them to survive. Most cells in the body may contain up to 1000 of these enzymes.

The bottom line is that enzymes are the reason we are able to digest the food we eat. Without enzymes food could not be digested and we would get no energy from the food.

There are three basic types of enzymes needed to sustain life. Two of these are produced within the body, and the third must be provided in the foods we eat.

These enzymes are:

1. Metabolic Enzymes

These are devoted to energy production in cells of our body, and further acts as detoxifying agents. Without these enzymes, we could not hear, see, feel, move or even think. These enzymes are produced within the walls of each cell; however several of our vital organs contribute towards their production.

2. Digestive Enzymes

This enzyme enables food to be broken down into its constituent nutrients. These nutrients can then be passed into the blood stream and what is not used is subsequently passed on as waste. Different enzymes apart from the one discussed earlier helps in the digestion of different types of foods, such as lactase discussed earlier.

3. Food enzymes

Food enzymes in raw foods help us to digest that particular kind of food, but not in the digestion of any other food. Cooking destroys the food enzymes and this must be taken seriously. Raw food or mildly cooked food is generally better in preserving these enzymes. Digestive enzymes produced in one body will usually allow cooked foods to be digested, but not to the degree possible once the food enzymes have been destroyed through overcooking. When food enzymes are destroyed through overcooking, it is harder for our digestive system to break down fats, protein and carbohydrates and the simple question is have you been overcooking your food?

Sometimes it can be better to ingest enzyme supplements, usually plant based enzymes, when suffering from certain digestive disorders. For instance pepsin is sometimes prescribed for people who appear to have difficulties digesting protein. Occasionally propain and bromelain are two plants based enzyme supplements often prescribed when the metabolic enzymes produced within the body requires help in fighting inflammation and there are other enzymes supplements for other conditions.

> **WHEN FOOD ENZYMES ARE DESTROYED THROUGH OVER COOKING, IT IS HARDER FOR OUR DIGESTIVE SYSTEM TO BREAK DOWN FATS, PROTEIN AND CARBOHYDRATES**

CHAPTER 3

3.00 <u>Fats</u>

It is quite obvious that most people tend to love fatty foods, especially foods like bacon, cheese, hamburger and many others. However irrespective of the fact that we all know that high fat diets are bad for our health, however the taste of these fatty foods seems to be irresistible for most people. In the United States and other European countries the diet seems to be 40% fat on average, most of which are saturated animal fats. Studies from different sectors over time have proven that these kinds of foods increase the risk for developing heart disease, and cancer plus other related disorders. Most of the foods people eat such as French fries, fried chicken, microwave popcorn, doughnuts, margarine, cookies and many others; contain an artery clogging fats, which can lead to type 2 diabetes, high cholesterol, cancer and other ailments.

> **FATTY FOODS SEEMS TO BE**
> **IRRESISTIBLE FOR MOST PEOPLE**

3.10 Bad fats

Saturated fats and Tran's fats are classed as bad fats because they increase our risk of heart disease, high blood pressure, cancer, diabetes and other related disorders.

From surface, saturated fats and Tran's fats tend to be solid at room temperature. What we must be concerned about is the level of intake of these fats, to prevent us from having the risk of developing the disorders associated with high consumption of these types of fats.

We must acknowledge that fat is a valuable energy source and carries fat solution vitamins necessary for proper growth and development, it also contributes towards the tastes associated with our food, but too much of this kind of fat is bad for our health. We must acknowledge that it is the total fat intake over time that eventually opens doors for chronic disorders, such as heart diseases, cancer, and diabetes and so on.

Some examples of bad fats;

Saturated fats
1. Ice cream
2. Cheese
3. Butter
4. Palm and coconut oil

5. Lard

6. Chicken with the skin

7. Whole fat dairy products (milk and cream)
8. High fat cuts of meat (pork lamb beef)

Tran's fats
1. Candy bars
2. Sticky margarine
3. Vegetable shortening
4. Fried foods such as French fries, fried chicken, chicken muggets, breaded fish.
5. Packaged snack foods Such as crackers, Microwave Popcorn
6. Commercially baked Pasties, cookies, cakes doughnuts, muffins.

IT IS THE TOTAL FAT INTAKE OVER TIME THAT EVENTUALLY OPEN DOORS FOR CHRONIC DISORDERS

3.20 Good Fats

Monounsaturated fats and polyunsaturated fats are known as the good fats because they are good for your heart, your cholesterol, and your overall health. For example, good fats have an obvious competition with bad fats, therefore is important to minimize the intake of Tran's fats and cholesterol (animal's fat) while consuming enough good fats. Also good fats raise your HDL or good cholesterol. One of the jobs of this High Density Lipoprotein (HDL) or good cholesterol is to grab your bad cholesterol, low density lipoprotein (LDL) and escort it to the liver where it is broken down and excreted. In the real sense, these good fats, attack some of the damages already done by the bad fats. This is good for people trying to get there cholesterol down and fight heart disease and other related disorders

Essential fatty acids (EFAS) are the goods fats well publicized all over the world today.

Essential fatty Acids (EFAS) are important fats that we cannot synthesize and must be obtained through diet. EFAS are long chain polyunsaturated fatty acids derived from linoleic, linolenic and oleic acids. They fall within three categories namely omega-3, omega 6 and omega 9

More about Essential Fatty Acids (EFAS)

1. Supports the cardiovascular, reproductive, immune and nervous system in our body. The human body needs these EFAs to manufacture and repair cells membranes, and allowing the cell to obtain maximum nutrition and expel harmful waste products from our body. The primary function of EFAS is the production of prostaglandins, which regulate body functions such as heart rate, blood pressure, blood clotting, fertility, conception, and further plays a vital part in the functioning of our immune system by regulating inflammation and encouraging our body to fight off infections. Essential fatty acids (EFAS) are also necessary for proper growth in children and fetuses and breast fed children; also require an adequate supply of EFAs, through their mother's diet.
2. The minimum healthy intake for both omega-3 and omega-6 acids, through diet per adult per day is 1.5 grams each. One table spoon of flaxseed oil can be sufficient or larger amounts of other omega-3 rich foods. We must bring to your attention that high heat destroys omega-3 acids and obtaining these acids by eating cooked foods is unlikely to provide sufficient amount.

3. Essential fatty acids (EFAs) omega 6/3 imbalance is linked with serious health problems such as heart attacks, cancer, insulin resistance asthma, lupus, schizophrenia, depression, accelerated aging, stroke, obesity, diabetes, arthritis, Alzheimer's disease, and many others.

Now let's look at these acids individually and the kind of foods they can be found in

A. Omega-3 (Linolenic acid)

Alpha linolenic acid (ALA) is the principal omega-3 fatty acid, which our body will convert into eicosapentaenoic acids (EPA) and later into docosahexaenic acid (DHA). EPA and the GLA synthesized from linoleic (omega-6) acid are later converted into hormone-like compounds known as eicosanoids, which aid in many bodily functions such as vital organ functions and intracellular activities.

Omega-3 are used in the formation of cell wall, making them supple and flexible and improving circulation and oxygen intake with proper red blood cells flexibility and functions.

Omega-3 deficiencies contribute to a number of disorders such as decreased memory and mental abilities, tingling sensation of the nerves, blood clots, reduced immune function, increased triglycerides and bad cholesterol (LDL) levels, impaired membrane functions, hypertension, irregular heartbeat, learning disorders, menopausal discomfort, itchiness on the front and the lower legs, growth malfunction in children, and so on.

Foods containing omega-3 (linolenic acids)

Flaxseed oil-It seems to contain the highest linoleic content of any food. Other foods that contain this acid are hempseed oil, walnuts, pumpkin seeds, Brazil nuts, sesame seeds, avocados, some dark green vegetables such as Kale, spinach, purslane, mustard greens, collards, canola oil, soybean oil, virgin oil, wheat germ oil, salmon, mackerel, sardines, and anchories, albacore tuna, and many others.

B. Omega-6 (Linoleic acid)

A healthy person with good nutrition will convert linoleic acid into garma linoleic acid (GLA), which will later be synthesized with EPA from the Omega-3 group into eicosanoids. Some omega-6 improve diabetic neuropathy, rheumatoid arthritis, skin disorders and aid in cancer treatment. Although most of us obtain sufficient linoleic acid, it is quite often not converted to GLA because of metabolic problems caused by diets rich in sugar, alcohol, and Tran's fats from processed foods, smoking, pollution, stress, aging, viral infections, diabetes and many others. It is advisable to eliminate some of these factors if possible, but others occasionally prefer to supplement with GLA rich foods such as borage oil, black current seed oil, or evening primrose oil.

Foods containing omega-6 (linoleic acid)

Flaxseed oil, flaxseed meal, hempseed oil, grape seed oil, pumpkin seed, pine nuts pistachio nuts, sunflower seeds (raw), olive oil, olives borage oil, evening primrose oil, blackcurrant seed oil, chestnut oil, chicken without the skin. You must avoid refined and hydrogenated versions of these foods. Others include, corn, safflower, sunflower, soybean, cottonseed oil.

C. Omega-9 (Oleic acid)

This acid is necessary, but on the balance of scale it is not an essential fatty acid because the human body can manufacture limited amount provided EPA's are present. Monounsaturated oleic acid lowers heart attack risks, arteriosclerosis and aids in cancer prevention.

Foods containing omega-9 (Oleic acid) are extra virgin and virgin olive oil, olives, avocados, peanuts, sesame seeds, pecans, pistachio nuts, cashews, hazel nuts, macadamia nuts etc. One to two table spoons of extra virgin or virgin oil per day should provide sufficient oleic acid for adults.

General advice on foods

1. High heat, light and oxygen destroy EFA's, therefore when consuming foods, try to avoid cooked or heated forms.
2. Never re-use any type of oil for cooking
3. Extra virgin olive oil or grapes seed oil are best recommend for cooking because they tend to withstand high heat better.

Monounsaturated fats	polyunsaturated fats
1. Olive oil	Soybean oil
2. Canola oil	Corn oil
3. Sunflower oil	Safflower oil
4. Peanut oil	Walnuts

5. Sesame oil
6. Avocado's
7. Olives
8. Nuts (Almonds, Peanuts)

   Cashews, Hazel nuts,
   Pecans, macadamia nuts.
9. Peanut butter

Sunflower, Sesame
Pumpkin seeds
Flaxseeds
Salmon, Tuna, Mackerel,
Sardines, herring, trout,
soymilk, Tofu.

**ESSENTIAL FATTY ACIDS (EFA'S)
OMEGA -3/6 IMBALACE IS LINKED
WITH SERIOUS HEALTH PROBLEM
SUCH AS HEART ATTACK**

3.30 Low fat foods

To benefit from low fat foods, it is obvious that we have to make some sacrifice around the dinner table. This means replacing high fat foods with their low fat equivalent.

Choice for low fat foods example

1. Olive oil, canola oil, safflower oil.
2. Water packed tuna, salmon, and sardines.
3. Peas, carrots, corn, mushrooms, peaches, asparagus, pineapple, pears.
4. Crushed tomatoes, tomato purees, tomato sauces (with no added salt).
5. Canned or dried black beans, pinto beans, chicken peas, kidney beans, navy beans, black eye beans, rice lentils, barley couscous, quinoa, kamuts.
6. Whole wheat, spaghetti, penne, lasagna sheets, and other noodles
7. Anchories, capers, pimientos, peppers, artichokes, pickles, sundried tomatoes, minced garlic.
8. Low fat, low sodium canned soups, and soup mixes, low sodium fat free broths.
9. Herbs, spices, seasoning, whole garlic, garlic paste, tomato paste, chili paste, bottled ginger, soy sauces, bottled marinades.
10. Low fat or fat free salad dressings and mayonnaise.
11. Whole grain bread, rolls and bagels, whole wheat flour, whole grain cereals such as oat meal, bran flakes, or low fat granola.
12. Cranberries, cherries, blueberries, and resins
13. Almonds, hazelnuts, walnuts, peanuts, pecans, pumpkin seeds, sunflower seeds, sesame seeds, puppy seeds, flax seeds,
14. Honey, molasses, maple syrup
15. Pretzels, low fat microwave popcorn, whole grain crackers, sugar free /fat free pudding and apple sauce.
16. Apples, bananas all raw
17. Chickens, broilers breast (meat only cooked or roasted)
18. Cheese cottage low fat
19. Fish, haddock, cooked dry heat

20. Fish roughly orange, cooked dry heat
21. Beef ground 95% lean meat/5% fat.

These lists are just some examples.

```
TO BENEFIT FROM LOW FAT FOODS, IT
IS OBVIOUS THAT WE HAVE TO MAKE
SOME SACRIFICES AROUND THE
DINNER TABLE
```

3.40 High fat foods

People are beginning to understand that there are certain foods to eat and others to avoid. While we acknowledge the foods that contribute to a healthy diet such as foods that are low in fat and cholesterol and high fiber foods such as whole grain foods, vegetables, fruits, foods with moderate amount of sugar and salt, calcium rich foods to meet a Childs daily calcium requirements, iron rich foods to meet our daily need for iron. However the truth is that some people are still obsessed with eating high fat foods especially with the advent of a lot of fast foods outfits. Of course we should all avoid a lot of high fat foods and high calories foods if we want to stay healthy, but sometimes our habits and the tasteful nature of these foods make them irresistible to us, and we must all try to draw some line at a certain stage of our life and start eating healthy.

A good approach is to first learn how to recognize foods that are high in fat by reading food labels. In general a food that is high in fat will usually have 13g or 20% daily value of requirement of fat per serving or more, while a low fat food will have in the region of 3g or 5% daily value of fat per serving or less.

Some typical high fat foods are

1. Chocolate candies
2. Cheese sauce
3. Ribs
4. Baked beans with franks
5. Spinach souffbaglé
6. Cheese Cake
7. Hash brown potatoes
8. All gratin potatoes
9. Potato salads
10. Homemade white sauce
11. Condensed milk (sweetened)
12. Pie (pecan, cherry, chocolate, crème etc)
13. Chicken pot pie
14. Ricotta cheese made with or part skim milk
15. Trail mix, especially varieties containing chocolates chips.
16. Beef, lamb, turkey and chicken with high fat.

High fat fast foods

1. Egg and sans eye biscuits
2. Double meat hamburgers and cheese burgers.
3. Tacos
4. Chicken fillet sandwiches
5. French fries
6. Milk shakes
7. Fish sandwiches with cheese
8. Croissant with egg, cheese and bacon
9. Tuna salad submarine sandwich
10. French toast sticks
11. Chicken pieces (fried nuggets or strips)
12. Nachos
13. Corn dogs
14. Enchiladas
15. Cold cuts submarine sandwich
16. Onions rings

It must be acknowledge that the level of these fats will depend on the serving sizes you eat. These are just some examples of the foods we should all look out for and consume to a minimum.

```
WE SHOULD AVOID A LOT OF HIGH
FAT FOODS AND HIGH CALORIE FOODS
IF WE WANT TO STAY HEALTHY
```

3.50 Reducing blood cholesterol and fats

Cholesterol is a fatty material usually made in the body from saturated fat in our diet. It plays an important role in cell function throughout the body and it is the building block of many essential steroid hormones. There are some good and bad cholesterol.

However if we have too much of the bad cholesterol in our blood stream, it increase our risk of developing coronary heart disease. Cholesterol uses the body's circulation as its road network and is carried through avenues consisting of proteins known as lipoprotein.

There are two main types, low density lipoprotein (LDL) which carries cholesterol from the liver to the cells, and the high-density lipoprotein (HDL) which returns excess cholesterol back to the liver.

The cause of coronary heart disease is the narrowing of the arteries that supply the heart from a gradual accumulation of fatty materials, a condition called atherosclerosis.

Atherosclerosis occurs when LDL cholesterol, the bad cholesterol is deposited on the walls of the coronary arteries, however HDL which is termed as the good cholesterol removes this cholesterol from the circulation and protects against coronary heart disease.

The bottom line is that the ratio of HDL and LDL in our blood stream is very vital and that we should all aim for a low LDL and a high HDL.

Good cholesterol level

The average blood cholesterol level of people living in United Kingdom is 5.8mmolL; this refers to 5.8 millimoles per liter of blood.

Cause of high cholesterol

The most common cause of high cholesterol is too much consumption of saturated fat in our diet, lack of physical exercise, and an inherited gene which tends to produce too much cholesterol called familial hypercholesterolemia.

Lowering our cholesterol level

To lower our cholesterol, we must cut down on the intake of all fats, especially saturated fats and eat more starchy foods. We should eat only fish which helps to raise healthy HDL cholesterol. Diet alone can usually reduce cholesterol by between 5 to 10 percent. Monounsaturated fats found in olive oil, rape seed oil, avocados, walnuts etc, tend to lower LDL cholesterol without lowering HDL cholesterol.

Top foods to lower your cholesterol

1. Oatmeal, oat bran and high fiber foods

   Oatmeal contains soluble fiber which reduces LDL. The soluble fiber can also be found in kidney beans, apples, pears, barley prunes etc. Soluble fiber can reduce the absorption of this bad LDL cholesterol into our blood stream. 5 to 10grams or more soluble fiber a day decreases our total LDL

2. Fish and omega-3 fatty acids

   Eating fatty fish is good for our heart because of its high level of omega 3 fatty acids which can reduce our blood pressure and the risk of developing blood clots. In people who have already experienced heart attack, fish oil or omega 3 fatty acids reduces the risk of sudden death. Most doctors recommend that we should eat at least two servings of fish a week and these can be found in mackerel, lake trout, herring, sardines, albacore, tuna, salmon, halibut etc. It is recommended that we should bake or grill the fish to avoid adding unhealthy fats. People who don't like fish can get small amounts of omega-3 fatty acids from foods such as ground flaxseed or canola oil or you can get omega-3 fish oil supplement.

3. Walnuts, almonds and other nuts

   Walnuts, almond and other nuts can reduce blood cholesterol. They are rich in polyunsaturated fatty acids. Walnuts also help to keep our blood vessels healthy. Eating about a handful of most nuts a day such as almonds, hazelnuts, peanuts, precons, walnuts, pistachio, can reduce your risk of heart disease, however you must ensure that the nuts are not salted or coated with sugar.

Medication

Medication is given if the cholesterol level remains too high despite dietary measures, and if the overall risk of heart disease is likely to be greater than 20% over a 10 years period.

A drug commonly use is called statins, they usually reduce LDL cholesterol by more than 20% and reduce the risk of dying from heart disease by around 25%. However they are not suitable for everyone and your doctor must be consulted. An alternative to statins, Ezetimibe has been developed, and your doctor should advice you more.

Ways to reduce fat

1. Red meat

Eat smaller portion of meat in your diet and larger quantities of beans, vegetables and eat lean cuts of meat and remove any visible fat.

2. Cheese

All hard and cream cheese is high in fat and you must reduce the portion of cheese in sauces and dishes. Eat low fat cheese such as edam, gonda, jar/sberg and cottage cheese.

3. Salads

Mayonnaise and salad creams contain a high proportion of fat. Make salad dressings with natural yogurts, herbs, spices, tomato juice, vinegar, and lemon juice. You can also use French dressing; make yours from lemon juice, organic olive oil, cider or wine vinegar, crushed garlic, and a tea spoon of readymade mustard. Put a mixture of green salad leaves, with a few walnuts, flaked toasted almonds, pumpkin seeds, apples and celery and mix in some French dressing.

4. Sandwiches

We must use small amount of margarine or butter or spread on one side of the bread only.

5. Milk

Take skimmed milk or skimmed milk powder

6. Fish

We should eat more of this delicacy such as tuna fish, risotto; salmon stir fry, or smoked mackerel with baked potatoes. These oily fish are high in good fats or essential fats. They are a good source of omega 3 and omega 6 fatty acids, which are essential for our body hormone level balance, thereby reducing inflammation in joints and produces elastic connective tissues which is an avenue for enhancing our skin.

7. Soups

Soften vegetables in splash of olive oil before making soups. Use a vegetable stock or add water and season the herbs, a dash of tamari or some shoyu. Tamari and shoyu are common in China; they add richness in soups without a trace of meat or fat and tend to be very good for a vegetarian dish.

8. Cream

Eat low fat yogurt instead of cream.

9. Poultry

Use chicken but remove the skin

10. Pastry

Avoid short crust cheese or flaky pastry. Use filo pastry on the top of a dish only. An alternative is a potato or an oat crumble.

> **THE RATE OF LDL AND HDL IN OUR BLOOD IS VERY VITAL AND WE SHOULD ALL AIM FOR A LOW LDL AND A HIGH HDL**

3.60   Bad and good foods

Bad foods

1. **Solid fats from land animals**

   We must limit these saturated fats. To absorb these land animals fats, we increase our production of cholesterol to make bile. Its re-intake from the bowel, if we lack vitamin C and fiber is what raises blood cholesterol that is the LDL.

2. **Trans partially hydrogenated and most deep fry oils**

   Common in most commercial fries, used for chips, chickens, shortenings, known to be tasty but toxic. There is no nutritional excuse to hydrogenate anything. They tend to lower good cholesterol (HDL) and raise their bad equivalent (LDL). About 40% of the fat in doughnuts fries, cookies, crackers, margarine etc, is Tran's fat. I doughnut + I fries = 10g of toxic missile, called Tran's fat. Not only does Tran's fat destroy our nutrients, but they also make them toxic.

3. **Flour (white refined) and flour made pasta.**

   The more finely ground the flour and the more boiled the noodle, the higher the glycemic index, which is not really healthy. They lack essential nutrients and are proven inferior to whole grain products. They are linked to increase heart disease. There rapid absorption causes fast changes in sugar/insulin balance, and eventually cell resistance to both, which eventually can result in adult diabetes.

In general, bad foods are most processed foods, which tend to contain a lot of sugar, salt, and fats. These tend to be fatty foods like, margarine, butter, cream, most cheese, fatty meat, sugar and sugary foods like cake, candies, ice cream, milk shakes, sugary drinks like soda, are also foods containing additives and colorings.

Other foods that are classed as bad include, junk foods, fast foods and take ways. The bottom line is to eat these kinds of foods in moderation or avoid them altogether.

Good foods

Almost any food that is fresh is a good choice, better still is fresh organic foods. In these categories, we have to look at oily fish, vegetables, fruits, oats and other fiber rich grains, pulses, beans, peas, some vegetable oils which are high in monounsaturated fats, such as olive and canola oil.

Some of the top choices are

1. **Mangoes**

   Just one cup supplies 100% of a day's vitamin C, one third of a day's vitamin A, a good dose of blood pressure lowering potassium and 3 gram of fiber.

2. **Sweet potatoes**

   They are high in carotenoids, vitamin C, Potassium and fiber.

3. **Unsweetened Greeks yogurt**

   Non-fat and contain a good amount of protein.

4. **Broccoli**

   It has lots of vitamin C, carotenoids, vitamin K and folic acid.

5. **Wild salmon**

   The Omega-3 fats in the fish can help reduce the risk of sudden death from heart attack.

6. **Crisp breads**

   Whole grain rye crackers like wasa, kavli, ryvita are loaded with fiber and are usually fat free.

7. **Garbanzo beans**

   All beans are good; they are all rich in protein, fiber, iron, magnesium, potassium, and zinc, but garbanzo beans stands out.

8. **Water melon**

   Contain a good dose of Vitamin A, and C plus potassium and lycopene. They are fat free with salt free calories.

9. **Leafy greens**

   These include kale, collards, spinach, turnip greens, mustard greens, Swiss chard etc. These are good sources of vitamin A, C and K, and folate, potassium, magnesium, calcium, iron, lutein, and fiber.

10. **Butter mint squash**

   A very good source of vitamin A, C and fiber.

11. **Oats and other fiber rich grain**

12. **Olive and canola oil**

IN GENERAL, BAD FOODS ARE MOST PROCESSED FOODS WHICH TEND TO CONTAIN A LOT OF SUGAR, FAT, AND SALT

3.70   Foods that make you look older

While we acknowledge the facts that we all want to look younger, however there are certain foods and things that can actually reverse the situation and make us look a lot older than our age.

1. Sugar

    Sweets and refined carbohydrates tend to increase our blood glucose levels, which interferes with the normal repair of collagen and elasticity and subsequently reflects on our looks. Therefore if we want to look great and receive all the compliments that go with it, we must limit the intake of sugar, especially sweets and refined carbohydrates.

2. Saturated fats

    Diets that are high in saturated fats tend to provide an avenue for increased inflammation and in so doing ages our skin.

3. Alcohol

    Alcohol tends to dehydrate our body, leaving our skin tight and dry. Our liver also releases skin aging free radicals as it metabolizes our alcohol intake.

> **DIETS HIGH IN SATURATED FAT
> TEND TO PROVIDE AN AVENUE FOR
> INCREASED INFLAMMATION**

3.80   <u>Foods that can make you look younger</u>

We all know that fresh fruits and vegetables are the key to improving our general health; clearer skin and bright youthful complexion, however combined with these are some other foods that can make us look a lot younger than our age.

Now below are some of these key foods if we want to maintain our youthful appearance. Nutrition researchers in Australia, Greece, and Sweden studied 450 people aged 70 and over to see if the foods they ate related to how wrinkly they looked. They found that the least wrinkled people mainly ate or drank the following foods.

1.   Legumes such as peas, beans, lentils, peanuts and altalfa.
2.   Vegetables
3.   Fish
4.   Tea
5.   Low fat milk products

And the more wrinkled people ate more full fat dairy foods such as butter, margarine, red meat, fizzy soft drinks, cakes, and pasties.

Antioxidants and the retardation of wrinkles

Studies in antioxidants suggest that they tend to retard wrinkles.

A research at Hebrew university faculty of Agriculture, food and Environmental quality science has found that a certain antioxidant fights wrinkles. Dr. Orit Bossi managed to isolate an antioxidant from plants that slows down the aging process.

She concluded that because some antioxidant oxidizes quickly, they lose their efficiency over time. But the antioxidant she researched on can withstand high temperature, is soluble in water, and does not oxidize easily. The conclusion is that they tend to stay effective over time and counters the breakdown of collagen fibers in the skin.

Antioxidants fight free radicals in our body that usually causes a breakdown of many body tissues including our skin. They include vitamin E, vitamin C, and the antioxidant EGCG in green tea.

In general, small amount of free radicals are less harmful to our body, however in situation of an excess free radicals due to our normal aging process or because of excessive exposure to ultra-violet radiation, the result is that the collagen and elastic fibers in our skin breakdown and it loses its elasticity resulting in the appearance of wrinkles, which make us look older.

Grapes and red wines prevention of aging

A compound called resveratrol, a natural compound found in red grapes, mulberries, peanuts and red wine can slow down the effects of aging while protecting our heart.

Further studies have found that mice that were fed with high-fat diet and were also given resveratrol lived longer than their counterparts that were deprived the compounds.

Resveratrol seems to offer protection against heart disease by acting as an antioxidant antimutagen and anti-inflammatory.

Holy basil

Holy basil is an Indian relative of basil plant, which is a herb commonly used in Indian medicine to treat headache, colds, stomach disorders, heart disorders and many others.

Researchers from Poona College of pharmacy in Maharashtra India studied holy basil to investigate its antioxidant and anti-aging properties. They concluded that it has some rejuvenating qualities and promotes a youthful state of physical and mental health by removing harmful molecules and protecting against damage caused by some free radicals in the heart, liver and brain. Further in this topic, it must be acknowledged that vitamin C, appear to play a vital role in our aging process and the appearance of wrinkles in our body. We must not forget the benefits of calcium, phosphorous, magnesium, zinc, iron, and resveretrol.

Further we must acknowledge that wrinkles tend to appear more in our body due to excessive exposure to the sun and as a result we must limit these exposures.

> **THE MORE WRINKLED PEOPLE ATE**
> **MORE FULL FAT DAIRY FOODS**

3.90 Foods and things that can cause body odor

We all know that body odors and bad breath appear to be an important area of concern in our lives. Some changes in our eating habits can go a long way to overcome these problems. Below are some foods that can make you stink, which we must look out for if we want to smell good.

1. Spices

Spices that have a high aroma when ingested will obviously produce sulfur gas, which is absorbed by the blood and eliminated through our lungs and pores of our skin. This causes bad breath and body odor. Some of these foods are garlic, onions, curry and many others. Now I am not saying that we should avoid the food or spices but to limit the amount of intake.

2. Red meat.

It usually takes a longer time to digest red meat. When undigested, food toxins and foul smelling gases are released, which usually causes perspiration odor.

3. Alcohol and caffeine

The reduction of the above, will obviously improve our smell and hygiene.

4. Processed foods and junk foods

Eating a lot of processed foods, that is high in salt, sugar, flour, hydrogenated oils, tends to rot in our stomach and produces body odor and bad breath.

5. Tobacco

Tobacco usually gives us bad breath. They also mix with other elements in our body and are discharged through the sweat glands which causes body odor which can last for days.

6. Fried

Fats and oils in foods that are fried and fatty foods become rancid over time and can cause digestive disorder, which can cause bad body odor.

7. Dairy products

Dairy products are rich protein and when broken down in our stomach can cause the escape of hydrogen sulfide and methyl mercaptan and can obviously cause some bad smell.

8. Low carbohydrate

Reducing the intake of carbohydrate in place of protein rich foods, can assist in burning fat in our body, but the process releases ketones into our blood stream that makes our sweat smell bad.

9. Choline

Foods that are high in choline usually contribute to a smelly sweat, such as fish. If you find it difficult to digest fish quickly, you will tend to smell fishy. Other foods that are applicable are egg, liver and nuts etc.

10. Trimethylamine

This is a genetic disorder which means that the body is unable to break down amino acids, which tends to produce a fishy body odor. Some of the foods that contain amino acids are seafood's, fish oil, eggs, liver, milk, nuts, soy products, broccoli etc.

To prevent body odor, we must drink a lot of water and consume foods containing fiber, fruits and low choline such as apples, strawberries, oranges, grapes, tomatoes, pineapples bananas, watermelon etc.

> **IF YOU FIND IT DIFFICULT TO DIGEST FISH QUICKLY, YOU WILL TEND TO SMELL FISHY**

3.100 <u>Healthy foods and some risk factors</u>

Though some of this food can add to our good health and well being, however we must realize some risk factors associated with these foods, and below are some good examples.

1. **Fish**

   While fish provides us with good protein and omega-3 fatty acids, we must acknowledge that some fish can put us at an increased risk for methyl/mercury poisoning. Most fish contains some form of contamination of mercury, particularly shark, sword fish, King mackerel, and tilefish register a considerable high level of mercury contamination. Smaller fish such as canned light tuna appear to have lower levels of mercury contamination. The issue here is that we must keep an open eye and know the kind of fish we consume.

2. **Baked beans**

   It is obvious that beans contain a lot of fiber and protein. But we must try not to soak them in a can of syrup that has a lot of sugar and as many soda. By doing this, we tend to destroy most of the health benefits. For better health benefits it is better to eat beans such as kidney beans rather than the baked variety.

3. **Protein bars**

   This tends to have a lot protein and vitamins, including fat and sugar. They are good for an occasional snack but not for your regular meals because they are not far off from a candy bar. We should be looking for a high quality protein instead.

4. **Low fat salad dressings**

   Fat usually tends to give our food that essential taste that appears to be irresistible. And when fat disappears, the taste in replaced with sugar or those potential cancer causing artificial sweetener.

5. **Bran muffins**

   Bran muffins are loaded with refined flour and processed sugar which tends to put us at some form of health risk.

6. **Fruits juice**

   100% fruit juice is packed with a considerable quantity of sugar to rot our teeth and also give us type 2 diabetes if we drink it a lot. The idea here is to limit our consumption.

7. Diet Soda

While we have lost the sugar contents of the drink, we have at the same time separated the sugar for a carcinogenic artificial sweetener. It is a lot better for us to try a sparkling water or low fat milk.

8. Yogurt

While the natural unsweetened yogurt provides us with good protein, calcium and increase our digestive health. However some are packed with fruits and corn syrup that can make us consume quite a lot of sugar. Besides there are also some Artery-clogging fats in a lot of these yogurts.

5. Granola

Most granola tend to be high in processed sugar and granola bars are not an exception, and we must avoid them.

6. Tofu

Tofu seems to be quite good but must be eaten in moderation because high consumption of soy has been shown to increase estrogen in males and has been linked to breast and cancer risk in females. It has been acknowledged that soy has the potential to alter reproductive and hormonal development. Some claim that unfermented soy contains a variety of toxic chemicals.

MOST FISH CONTAINS SOME FORM OF CONTAMINATION OF MERCURY

CHAPTER 4

4.00 Eating habits

It is quite obvious that eating habits usually has some considerable impact in our life's and well being. Some of these habits can either be good or bad. Good eating habits usually help us lose weight, feel more energetic and put us at a reduced risk of illness and subsequently extend our life span. On the other hand, bad eating habits will usually create room for illness, fatigue and reduced life span.

The truth is that bad eating habits tends to eat away our health, they tend to make us look fat, sluggish and unhealthy. Bad eating habit seems to be a choice of ignorance.

We all want to look good and vibrant and in subsequent headings, we will have to explore more in details about our eating habits which can be either good or bad.

> **BAD EATING HABITS SEEM TO BE A CHOICE OF IGNORANCE**

4.10   Good eating habits

Good eating habits come with commitments and your effort including discipline. Below are some of these goods eating habits;

1. **Always enjoy your breakfast instead of skipping it**

   The skipping of breakfast can throw our metabolism off for hours. We must eat morning meals, and must stay away from pasties, pancakes, waffles and other super sweet starchy heavy foods. A good idea is to concentrate on eating whole grain breads or cereals, low fat protein sources like peanut butter, lean meats, fish, low fat dairy products like skim milk, low fat yogurt, low fat cheese or either fresh fruits or 100% fruit juice.

2. **Eat meals on a table and not on the run**

   You must endeavor to respect your dinner time. Why not form the habit of always eating on a table, rather than eating while driving or working. This will usually encourage you to eat more because it is unlikely you will be satisfied.

3. **You must drink enough water**

   Why not form the habit of drinking enough water during your meal to aid your digestive system. Do not form the habit of eating without water. It's best to drink water after eating.

4. **Try to have some healthy snack food**

   Instead of going to a vending machine for a candy bar to stop your mid afternoon hunger, why not try for some low salt nuts or fresh fruits like orange, bananas, apples etc.

5. **Slow down your eating**

   The truth is that if you take your time to eat, you will eat and enjoy it more.

6. **Limit alcohol to1-2 drink per day**

   This will assist you to avoid unrealistic weight gain and other related health problems associated with alcohol.

7. **Avoid talking too much while eating**

   The simple logic is to concentrate and enjoy your meal and talk less. How often have we all experience some unnecessary coughing due to excessive talking and eating.

8. <u>Do not over eat</u>

You should try not to form the habit of eating everything on your plate. If you are full, stop eating. If you are the type that dislikes wasting foods, why not put the balance in you fridge for another day.

4.20 <u>Bad eating habits</u>

1. Eating on the run
2. Using food to ease stress
3. Overeating to prevent wastage of food
4. Late night eating
5. Skipping meals
6. Binging
7. Eating while working
8. Eating too fast
9. Eating without water or enough water
10. Drinking alcohol on an empty stomach
11. Starving Yourself

1. <u>Eating on the run</u>

Having a hectic life style will usually not allow you to settle down and prepare your meal or even sit down to eat. You might even be prone to eating in the car while driving or eating while walking. This means you will not have time to pay good attention to your diet. And eating this way will always mean that you will eat more and get fat and unhealthy.

2. <u>Using food to ease stress</u>

I know that all those hectic days at work can lead to stress and occasionally the only way out is to eat more. Also some men or women tend to eat more when they experience a failed relationship, but this is not the answer. It will lead to weight gain and other health problems.

3. <u>Over eating to prevent wastage of food</u>

You don't have to finish all the food on your plate when you are full. Try to keep the balance in your fridge for another day.

4. <u>Late might eating</u>

This will usually put you right to sleep and usually causes weight gain. If you eat large meal that are high in carbohydrate before your body goes to rest, chances is that your body will not burn them all and when your body goes into repair and store mode because you are not active enough, your body may turn the food into fat.

5. **Skipping meals**

   Skipping meals is a bad one especially breakfast, because the breakfast usually gives us a boost of energy and helps us clear the fog out of our brain. Also skipping meals can create some health disorders such as ulcers, because the acid in our stomach might start attacking our stomach walls, which if prolonged can create some stomach wounds known as ulcer. Also if we don't eat regularly, our hunger increases and we may also experience a drop in sugar level, making us feel tired.

6. **Binging**

   We all know that food binging come in form of fatty snacks like chips, pizza, cookies, candy bars etc. This is bad for us.

7. **Eating while working**

   This will obviously lead to over eating and spilling of foods all over. This habit will make you less full and will eventually lead to overeating later.

8. **Eating too fast**

   Eating too fast will obviously make you eat more and gain more weight. You will most likely choke in between these meals and cough more.

9. **Eating without water or enough water**

   I believe the digestive system needs more of this water to work properly and not having water at all is even worst.

10. **Drinking alcohol on an empty stomach**

    Have a few drinks on an empty stomach and you will be eating up everything on sight in an attempt to get your glucose level higher. Now ask yourself why? This is because our body sees alcohol as poison and tries to clear it from our body as quickly as possible thereby interrupting our normal glucose production and hence the low blood sugar will make us more hungry and hence we eat more.

11. **Starving yourself**

    Surprisingly, our bodies' first reaction to starvation is weight gain through the storage of fat. When you don't eat for long periods of time, your body thinks it needs to store calories as fat because it does not know when the chance to eat will come again and the fat remains with you.

SKIPPING MEALS CAN CREATE SOME HEALTH DISORDERS SUCH AS ULCER

4.30   Tips to healthy eating

1.   Eat a variety of nutrient rich foods

We usually require more than 40 different nutrients for good health and no single food provides for these nutrients. Our daily food selection must include bread and other whole grain products, fruits, vegetables, dairy products, poultry, fish, meat, and other protein foods. Your food intake will depend on your calories needs for instance, if you intend to be more active for the day, your calories intake can be higher.

2.   Eat plenty of whole grains fruits and vegetables

We tend to eat less of these foods which must put right.

3.   Maintain a healthy weight

The weight that is right for us depends on many factors such as sex, age, height and heredity. We must acknowledge that excess body fat increase our chances of high blood pressure, heart disease, strokes, diabetes, cancer and other related disorders. Also being too skinny can increase our risk for osteoporosis, menstrual irregularities and other related problems.

4.   Eat regular meals

You must avoid skipping meals; this can lead to ulcer and out of control hunger.

5.   Eat moderate portion of foods

Do not try to finish the whole food in your plate if you are full. Try to select moderate portions.

6.   Drink enough water

You must enjoy your food with water and avoid eating without water. Lack of water in our body leads to dehydration. If your urine tends to be very yellowish in color, it is most likely you haven't been drinking enough water. You must then top up even if you are not tasty.

7.   Reduce but don't eliminate certain foods

If your best foods tend to be high in fat, salt or sugar, the important thing is to minimize on their intake and how often you eat them. If you think you have exceeded certain limits, follow it up with some exercises to burn off some fats.

8. Make changes gradually

Changing too fast in your diet can lead to failure. Remedy deficiencies with modest change that can lead to improved lifelong eating habits pattern.

9. Balance your food choices

For instance, if you tend to eat food high in fat, salt, and sugar, balance it with other foods low in fat, salt and sugar.

10. Know your diet pit falls

To make positive changes in your eating pattern, you must first establish what is wrong with them. It is important for you to write down everything you eat over a one week period and then check on your intake in form of appraisal, such as whether you take a lot of saturated fats, salts, sugar, low water, inadequate fruits, vegetables, including whole grains and cereals and then make the relevant amendments for a more balanced diet.

Access how you feel when you consume these foods to enable you to know the ones to avoid or perhaps to look for a better substitute.

> **IF YOUR URINE TENDS TO BE YELLOWISH IN COLOUR, IT IS MOST LIKELY THAT YOU HAVEN'T BEEN DRINKING ENOUGH WATER**

4.40   Tips for a healthy looking skin

1.   Eat a well balanced diet

To look healthy, our skin requires a regular and well balanced supply of nutrients. We must try to eat at least five portions of fresh vegetables or fruits every day, which will be quite simple if we have three pieces as desert or snacks plus a salad or vegetable dish with two meals.

2.   Drink a lot of water

One of the many causes of a skin that looks tired is dehydration both on the surface and throughout our body. We must learn to re-hydrate our body by drinking about six glasses or more of water per day. This should be ideally taken plain or lightly flavored, but unsweetened.

3.   Cut down on the intake of coffee, hot chocolates and cola type drinks and certain teas.

These types of drinks make our skin to suffer from spots and greasy skin. This is because these drinks contain caffeine which prevents our body from making good use of our diet. We must limit our coffee intake to no more than three cups per day, which includes tea and other caffeine containing drinks.

4.   Keep the drinking of alcohol to a minimum

Drinking a lot of alcohol can cause certain skin problem such as split veins. We should maintain the recommended 21 units per week. A unit is equivalent to a glass of wine. Some women have a skin allergy to some alcoholic drinks, which usually show up as hives.

Hives are little itchy red spots that appear under the surface of the skin and make it feel hot and sensitive. They are occasionally called nettle rash. The most common allergic reaction to salicylates substances can occur naturally in some foods, such as grapes, banana's, beans, strawberries and other berry products. If you get a rash after eating any of these foods, beers can affect you in the same manner since bear is high in salicylates. Instead you must choose wine, gin, vodka or whisky.

5. <u>Try to give up smoking.</u>

Nicotine does not help us keep a healthy skin. They tend to attack the blood vessels that feed the skin.

> **DRINKS CONTAINING CAFFEINE PREVENTS OUR BODY FROM MAKING GOOD USE OF OUR DIET**

4.50   Steps to changing bad eating habits

Changing bad eating habits is not a matter of for casual approach; you must acknowledge your bad habits and then do something about it. This requires total commitment and effort from your part.

It is not just embarking on your journey and then backing off at the midway stage.

You must look for what you want and then put together a good strategy that will work for you.

You must be prepared to do something about those eating cravings and the way you do it. For instance some people enjoy eating their food with only alcohol instead of water. If this habit has become part of you, perhaps you have to gradually adjust this life style. Perhaps having some water and a little bit of alcohol until you finally reach your goal of more of the water.

To change these bad eating habits, you must look at the following steps below

1. Find out what triggers your bad eating habits and then make an effort to break the chain. If for instance the vending machine at your work place encourages you to eat in an unrealistic way and time, why not avoid going through that route or perhaps ensure you don't have any loose change.
2. Why not give yourself some form of task or discipline whenever you get the urge to eat something in an unrealistic time or place. Perhaps condition yourself to wait just a little longer say 20 minutes. If you are not really hungry you will find out that you will tend to move on to other things until the ideal eating time becomes necessary.
3. Some people tend to eat unrealistically at parties and functions, occasionally while standing up and talking in most instances. Over time this habit tends to become part of them. If you are in this bracket of party animals, perhaps it is better to have a snack before going to the party and decide ahead of programme how many drinks you intend to have.
4. You must start with the easiest changes first, to give you more confidence to tackle the more difficulty ones.
5. State exactly what you want to achieve, for instance minimizing the intake of alcohol, must not eat after 9pm, must minimize food intake before bedtime etc.

6. Assess whether this is achievable and realistic.

7. Check whether perhaps certain people are involved in your bad habit by reviewing your day to day activity and then gradually look for a better solution to the problem.

8. Keep track of your progress and then review your program against your original plan.

9. Make any relevant changes necessary to keep you in track with you original goals.

While I acknowledge that old habits are not easy to break, however with considerable effort and determination we can always comes out on top.

> **SOME PEOPLE ENJOY THERE FOOD MORE WITH ONLY ALCOHOL, INSTEAD OF WATER**

4.60   How to lose belly fat

We all want to have that fantastic flat stomach that usually comes with a lot of compliments, but achieving this doesn't come easy for most people. We all know the added advantage of our exercise which helps us reduce stress and insulin levels and subsequently reduce the presence of cortisol, a hormone that accounts for more belly fat deposits. Cutting stress in our life, accounts for an indirect cut in belly fat in our body.

The way our body distribute fat in our body is beyond control and can be through our heredity gene, but what matters most is the level of our overall body fat which we must all try to lower and in so doing there wouldn't be much fat to deposit in the first instance.

Many women tend to gain more weight in their belly as they get older especially after menopause, when the body fat distribution changes and less fat goes to the arm, legs, hips, while more fat goes to the midsection. In some instances, we can experience a wider waistline, even though our weight remains static.

On the acknowledgement of all these points, below are some good ideas to lose belly fat.

1. **Exercise**
   Aerobic exercise will usually encourage the loss of fat all over our body including our belly. We must concentrate on calories burning exercises, instead of only sit ups and crunches if we want to lose belly fat. It is obvious that if our abdominal muscles are covered in fat, we will struggle trying to have that six pack and the key approach is the aerobic exercise.

2. Combine aerobic exercise with resistance training for better results in burning belly fat. Combining cardiovascular (aerobic) exercise, with some resistance training, will always do better in reducing our belly fat. Try using free weights exercise machines or resistance bands.

3. Reduction in calorie consumption. To lose belly fat, you must restrict your calories intake. If you tend to overeat, try reducing some of those calories and then continue your normal exercise.

4. You must get rid of refined grains for whole grains. Research shows that people who ate all whole grains, combined with five servings of fruits and vegetables,

three servings of low fat dairy products and two servings of lean meat, fish or poultry, lost more belly fat when compared with people who ate the same diet but with all refined grains. A diet high in whole grains alters the glucose and insulin response in our body which tends to increase the melting of visceral fat, that deep layer of fat is easier to burn than the subcutaneous fat under our skin.

5. Try eating the good fats

These includes fats with high ratio of monounsaturated fats such as avocados, nuts, soybeans, which can reduce the buildup of these belly fats. We must also acknowledge that Trans fats which are saturated fats, such as margarines, crackers, cookies, and things made with partially hydrogenated oils etc can result in more belly fats deposits.

6. Eat more of fiber

Soluble fibers such as apples, oats, cherries, lowers insulin levels, which usually increases the burning of visceral belly fat. When you eat fruits such as apples and potatoes, do not peel the skin off because all the fibers are there.

7. Learn to take in the region of 10,000 steps a day.

The more steps you take daily, the more in the reduction of belly fat. Don't just sit around all the time asking people to do things for you. Get up and take more steps to add to the reduction of your belly fat.

8. Motivate yourself by understanding the risk associated with belly fat and fat generally. Belly fat is linked with cardiovascular diseases, diabetes, cancer and other disorders. It is usually the deepest layer of the belly fat, the fat you can't see or grab that usually opens the doors to health risk. This is because the visceral fat cells produce hormones and other substances that can affect our health for instance, increased insulin resistance and/or breast cancer possibility. The truth is that belly fats are located right next to some vital organs and can drain into them putting us at some health risk. For instance, fat next to the liver, drains into it thereby causing a fatty liver and hence a risk factor for insulin resistance and hence a possibility for type 2 diabetes.

9. In reality a measurement of waist line of over 35 inches for women and over 40 inches for men are considered being unhealthy.

> **BELLY FAT ARE LOCATED RIGHT NEXT TO SOME VITAL ORGANS AND CAN DRAIN INTO THEM PUTTING US AT SOME HEALTH RISK**

4.70 <u>The power of what you eat and infections</u>

Infection is classed as any invasion of the body by disease causing micro organisms (germs) such as bacteria or virus. Many areas of our body are usually inhibited by micro organisms, but disease tends to develop when our body's defense system is faulty or the micro organisms move from their natural position to another area in our body. Other disease causing micro organisms usually enter our body through food, air, water, and contact with infected persons, environment, insects and animals etc.

Micro organisms enter the body through our skin, nose, mouth, ears, the intestinal or urinary tracts, anus and other body openings. In order to fight off these infections, the strength of our immune system is very vital. If you have a general poor nutrition, it significantly increases your chances of developing infection and diseases while the reverse will be the case if you embark on a balanced diet usually low in fat and high in fiber plus all relevant vitamins and minerals which enhances the immune response to infection and diseases.

In general some of the steps below will go a long way in helping us reduce infections.

1. Consume a low fat, high fiber, nutrient dense diet.
2. Your diet should contain a variety of fruits, vegetables, whole grain breads and cereals, cooked dried beans and peas.
3. Your diet should be low in sugar and refined and convenience foods.
4. A multiple vitamin minerals supplement that supplies up to 100% recommended dietary allowance for all vitamins and minerals should and be taken daily when your diet is not optimal.
5. Ensure you do regular exercise and stress management and control is recommended.
6. Minimize on the intake of alcohol and tobacco.
7. If necessary use your doctor's recommended antibiotic medication, and compliance to the doses.
8. You must ensure that you consume 6-8 glasses of water daily. Unless you are on certain medication, yellowish urine indicates that you probably need to top up the water level in your body.
9. Ensure that you have adequate level of sleep.

10. Maintain good environmental sanitation and avoid exposing your body to insects and animals that transmit diseases.

11. Avoid blood contact with infected people.

> **IF YOU HAVE A GENERAL POOR NUTRITION, IT SIGNIFICANTLY INCREASES YOUR CHANCES OF DEVELOPING INFECTIONS AND DISEASES**

4.80   <u>Other tips to stop you getting sick</u>

While we have to acknowledge that no one person is the same, the fact is that the majority of my readers will get better result from some of these tips. Now let's first of all look at the most common infection we all seem to experience all the time. But let us first look at this notion that seem to acknowledge that warm temperatures decreases sickness and the winter season tends to increase these ailments particularly flu and cold.

However studies have shown that what really matters here is the strength of the sun rays during these periods and how much vitamin D our body produces due to the UVB rays on our skin.

There are two theories most people tend to come across with the manifestation of more colds, flu and sicknesses during winter seasons.

1. The first is to do with most people keeping indoors during the winter months and are subsequently exposed to more germs within the enclosed building. But this theory will probably not hold any weight because people tend to go to work during this period and are still at their work place during the working hours.
2. Theory 2 seems to provide the best answer because people get sick more in the winter because of considerable reduction in their body's production of vitamin D which is directly responsible for how strong our immune system is.

The bottom line is that the sun rays tends to be low during the winter months which accounts for the considerable reduction in the vitamin D level in our body and subsequently reduces our immunity. The sunlight and Vitamin D levels are very good for the immune system and hormone production and balance. In reality, the reduction of sunlight and vitamin D is what is actually causing most people to get sick during the winter months.

Now how can we boost our immune system so that we can fight off diseases? Besides the advice already shown in paragraph 4.70. Here are some of the tips that can work for you,

1. The most important of this tip is the intake of vitamin D through diet. If you find that your diet falls short of this vitamins, why not go for some supplements.

You can get your vitamin D level tested and a good result will be between 40-70 ng/ml. Keep an eye on your vitamin D level especially during the winter months so that you don't have it dangerously low which can inhibit your immune system and hormone balance which subsequently leads to regular colds and hormone problems.

Vitamin D3 from either cold liver oil or an oil based D3 supplement are better options, however it is best to get vitamin D from the sun but do not over expose yourself.

2. Garlic

Garlic goes back thousands of years for treatment of sicknesses and recent studies shows that it boosts our immune system, aged garlic pills, whole garlic in food or garlic capsules will all do. If you feel a possible cold, flu or sickness within yourself, try loading garlic into your meals and take a few more garlic capsules for the period.

3. Kombucha tea (or other sources of probiotics)

This tea contains billions of friendly gut organism (probiotics) which helps to strengthen our immune system by increasing the levels of good organisms in our gut. We must acknowledge that 70% of our immune system lies in our gut flora and these organisms will protect us against pathogens and sickness.

You can also get beneficial probiotics from fermented foods such as sauer kraut (non-canned), yogurt kimchi etc. You can also take probiotic supplement drink called athletic greens.

4. Green tea

Green tea and chamomile tea tends to boost our immune system. They are also loaded with powerful antioxidants. Besides this tea, you can also drink other teas such as roobois tea, which is even higher in antioxidants than green tea.

5. Increase on antioxidants intake

An increase in antioxidant if you are having a sign of sickness will considerably boost your immune system. Some of the antioxidant rich foods are berries, teas, unsweetened cocoa, tomatoes, spirulina, chia seeds etc.

6. Exercise

A light exercise is very necessary if you feel a sign of sickness. Don't embark on a full workout because this will force your body to do a lot of recovery. It is also a good idea to go outside after your exercise for some fresh air and getting your body circulation system going properly and hence fighting off the sickness.

7. Avoid all processed foods and sweetened soft drinks.

   When you have a sign of sickness try not to overload your body with processed foods, fried foods, high fructose corn syrup, refined sugar and chemical additives which will force your body to do extra work to deal with all these junk foods and the internal inflammation that they can cause in our body. We should be eating foods that are meant to digest more efficiently in our body such as fruits, vegetables, eggs, nuts, seeds, and other easy digesting foods.

MOST PEOPLE GET SICK MORE IN THE WINTER BECAUSE OF CONSIDERABLE REDUCTION IN THEIR BODY'S PRODUCTION OF VITAMIN D

4.90   Acne pimple and diet

Acne is an inflammatory disease of the oil producing sebaceous glands of the skin. In most occasions it seems to manifest during puberty. Certain foods seems to encourage the manifestation of acne and some of these foods are chocolate, soft drinks, sugar, greasy foods, nuts, milk and salt etc.

If you are prone to acne, you must limit the intake of some of these foods or be careful in the selection of them.

Prevention

1. Ensure you thoroughly clean your skin daily to keep it free from dirt and oil.
2. Some doctors recommend zinc supplement for an effective treatment. Zinc usually maintains normal blood levels of vitamin A and plays a part in the normal functioning of the oil producing glands in the skin.
3. Antibiotics such as tetracycline seems to reduce the numbers of bacteria that break down the plugged oils and have been successful for some people, however a specialist seems to be the best answer.
4. A low fat high fiber nutrient dense diet sufficient in all vitamins and minerals and low in sugar and refined and convenience foods should be consumed.

> **CERTAIN FOODS SEEMS TO ENCOURAGE THE MANIFESTATION OF ACNE**

CHAPTER 5

5.00 Nutrients that can make us look a lot younger than our age

Studies have proved that antioxidants such as vitamin A, C, and E act like nature preservatives, which tend to slow or reverse the aging process. William pryor, professor of chemistry and biochemistry and director of the biodynamic institute at Louisiana State University, has found that certain nutrients are very good in reducing the incident of disease by about 50% and agrees that nutrition is a new form of medicine. Certain nutrients tend to make us look a lot younger than our age, and below are some of them.

1. **Beta-carotene**

   This antioxidant is the most potent time defying nutrient. Our body usually converts this antioxidant into a form of vitamin A. A plant form of Vitamin A tends to protect our body from cancer, heart disease, strokes and maintains good vision and keeps our skin looking young and healthy.

   Important sources of beta-carotene are dark green vegetables, carrots, cantaloupe, melon, apricots, spinach, broccoli, pumpkin, sweet potatoes, cabbage etc.

2. **Vitamin E**

   This antioxidant is known for foiling free radicals, chemicals that occur naturally in the body which tends to cause the death of healthy cells in our body. Vitamin E soaks up free radicals and protects our cells from damage. Vitamin E further reduces the risk of coronary heart disease and angina which is a severe pain in the heart muscles, which occurs when the heart doesn't receive enough oxygen and energy. Vitamin E helps to keep our blood from clotting easily and allows a smooth flow through the narrow coronary arteries. It also boosts our immune system and protects against cataract and cancer.

   Some good sources of vitamin E are dark green leafy vegetables, nuts such as almonds, peanuts, cashew nuts, palm nuts, coconuts, sweet potatoes, vegetable oils, wheat germs, and whole grains.

3. Vitamin C

This antioxidant boosts high-density lipoprotein (HDL) cholesterol, which is the good cholesterol, which prevents clogged arteries and puts the break on low density lipoprotein (LDL), the cholesterol which causes the blockage of arteries, which tend to lead to heart attack. Vitamin C also boost the immune system, guards against cancer, keeps the gums and teeth healthy, prevent eye cataracts, speeds the healing of wound, prevents asthma, and prevents infertility in men by maintaining sperm quality. Some sources of vitamin C are tomatoes, strawberries papaya, citrus fruits, broccoli, cantaloupes, water melon, red and green peppers etc.

4. Selenium

Selenium works as an anti-aging nutrient and helps to produce a special enzyme which in turn transforms certain free radicals into harmless water. This leads to a healthy immune system, and decreases the risks of diseases such as heart disease, strokes, cancer etc. Some good source of selenium are broccoli, celery, cucumbers, lobster, mushrooms, whole grains cereals and breads.

5. Zinc

Zinc is a part of an enzyme that protects our cells against free radicals. Our body depends on a steady supply of this mineral to keep our immune system healthy. Zinc assist in the healing of wounds, by assisting in the manufacture of new cells. Some good sources of zinc are lean beef, liver, poultry, fish, oysters, legumes, nuts etc.

6. Calcium

Calcium contributes for strong bones and help to increase our muscle power and nerve functions. It is always necessary to ensure you get enough calcium and for women, it is even more important because women are usually at risk of losing bone tissues, which can lead to a brittle bone condition called osteoporosis. Also calcium aids in preventing premenstrual symptoms such as irritability, anxiousness, depression, cramps, headaches, backaches etc. Some good sources of calcium are low fat and non fat milk and dairy products, broccoli, green leafy vegetables and legumes such as pinto beans etc.

7. Iron

Iron tends to operate in every part of our body and provides the body with oxygen needed for metabolism. Women who do not consume enough iron tends to suffer from anemia a condition characterized by feeling of extreme fatigue, headache, body chills, which can be due to lose of blood due to heavy period in women. Some good source of iron are Dark meat, poultry, lean meats, fish, iron fortified cereals and legumes.

8. Vitamin B6

This vitamin tends to keep our mind sharp and also improve our immune system. But vitamin B6 can be toxic in high doses and your doctor must be consulted for any supplements of vitamin B6. Some sources of vitamin B6 are bananas, plantain, chicken, fish, lean pork, oats and whole wheat products, peanut, soybeans, whole grain etc.

9. Vitamin B12

This vitamin sharpens our mind, keeps our energy reserves high, and is good for our joints. Our body needs a reasonable proportion of this vitamin; however we must take care in the consumption of alcohol which can hinder its absorption. Certain medications can also hinder its absorption. Some sources of vitamin B12 are eggs; learn meat, liver of beef, fish, low fat and non fat dairy products.

10. Water

Water tends to rank very high in most essential nutrients for a healthy looking body and also for healthy living. We tend to lose two to three pints every day on average and sometimes more. People tend not to drink enough to replace the water we lose from our body. We need between 6-8 glasses of water every day to keep our body organs functional.

Poor water intake exposes our kidney to a lot of stress. If we consume little water our skin will eventually become dry and wrinkly.

> **CERTAIN NUTRIENTS TEND TO
> MAKE US LOOK A LOT
> YOUNGER THAN OUR AGE**

5.10   Ten tips for an energizing life style

1. During breakfast, eat at least one serving of protein rich food, such as legumes, meat or low fat dairy products and at least two servings of fruits, vegetables and grains.

2. Limit the consumption of caffeinated beverages to three serving or less. Ensure that you don't drink tea and coffee with meals.

3. Ensure that you don't consume sugar alone and try to cut sugar intake down to a maximum of 10 percent of your total calories.

4. Eat several small meals and snacks approximately every four hours.

5. Eat a reasonable size low fat lunch that contains a mixture of protein and carbohydrates.

6. If you really enjoy carbohydrate and crave for it, plan a carbohydrate rich snack for your low energy period of the day.

7. Ensure you do not over eat in the evening and avoid too much snacking after dinner.

8. Avoid severe calorie restricted diets. This will usually affect your health in terms of trouble concentrating, impaired judgment, fatigue, poor memory etc.

9. Drink at least 6-8 glasses of water daily, low consumption will lead to dehydration and fatigue.

10. Avoid tobacco and limit your alcohol consumption. Tobacco is bad for your lungs and health and alcohol dehydrates the cells and suppresses the nervous system.

**TOBACCO IS BAD FOR YOUR
LUNGS AND HEALTH**

5.20 Ten ways to ease your tension

1. Watch your favorite film and listen to your favorite music. Try to choose the films that tend to make you laugh more or the music that brings back good memories. For me a comedy film tends to work.

2. Try to remember certain good and pleasant times in your life. You can even bring out some of those old pictures that tend to bring back good memories, and spend time thinking through them.

3. Breath easy

   Deep breathing is one of the simplest and good for stress management. According to Dean Ornish, president and director of preventive medicine research institute in Sausalito California, breathing deeply works by infusing the blood with extra oxygen thus cause the body to release endorphins, our body's natural tranquilizing hormones.

4. Take a walk

   When we are stressed, our body releases adrenalin to prepare our body to fight or flee. To get rid of the excess adrenalin we need to get moving and sitting on your favorite chair will only make things worse. Walking immediately assists in dissipating this chemical.

5. Think of what gives you that feeling of peace, perhaps the thought of trees, waves in the sea, your child, your wedding day, and your favorite holidays.

6. Get on the phone with your favorite friends, perhaps the one that make you laugh the most. Get into some interesting jokes if you can.

7. Undertake some light exercise, perhaps cycling etc.

8. Soak away your tension or stress with a warm bath, which will cool and relax your muscle and brain.

9. Rely on God

   Find a cool place and pray. Talk to God in your own way and believe that your God, will do wonders. You must have faith.

10. Confide in a good friend or family member. Don't sit around overhauling your problems or stress on your own, remember a problem shared is a problem solved.

```
BRING OUT SOME OF THOSE OLD
PICTURES THAT TENDS TO
BRING BACK GOOD MEMORIES
```

5.30 Tips to make you sleep well

1. **Think about what you eat**

   If you tend to over eat before going to bed, that will make you feel uncomfortable and subsequently harder to have a good night sleep. You must also think about the foods you are allergic to, for instance some people tend to avoid certain gassy foods such as beans before bed time.

2. **Avoid the intake of alcohol and caffeine**

   Do not drink caffeinated beverages before bed, and drinking too much alcohol before bed will result in poor quality sleep.

3. **Relax your body and mind**

   Try to wind down with a warm bath or bubble bath, and perhaps some kind of soft music or good book. You will fall asleep faster with this approach and sleep better.

4. **Keep a regular sleeping pattern**

   Ensure that you fall asleep and wake up roughly the same time every day; this will help set your biological clock properly.

5. **Before you go to bed, put your mobile phone on silent**

   Receiving unnecessary calls before your bed time or waking up to answer calls in between your sleep will result in poor quality sleep and can amount to some health problems such as headaches the next day and stress etc.

6. **Stop smoking**

   Nicotine is a stimulant that tends to affect our sleep.

7. **Ensure that your bed in comfortable**

   You bedroom must be the place you feel very relaxed, keep the light low, remove the television if you tend to be glued to it, and very important, ensure that your bed and pillow is comfortable.

8. <u>Forget about your troubles</u>

When going to bed try not to dwell on your troubles. It will tend to stimulate your brain and make sleep harder to come by. Think more about things that will make you more relaxed and happy. If you want, you can read some form of novel, and you can play some mild music, but keep the music volume low.

> **YOU MUST ALSO THINK ABOUT THE FOODS YOU ARE ALLERGIC TO**

5.40 <u>**Tips to avoid premature aging**</u>

The American Academy of Dermatology, define photo aging as damage to the skin caused by intense and chronic exposure to sun light. Photo aging is what causes those wrinkles, age spots and other unwelcomed pigmentations as we get older, which causes the skin to look rough and weathered.

The skin has a role to protect the body from various types of interference and external stimuli. This protection is achieved in a number of ways such as the formation of continuous layer of horn (Keratimization and release of epidermal cells that are already dead), respiration and body temperature regulation, the production of sebum and sweat ointment of skin, and to protect the formation of melanin, protection of the skin against the suns ultraviolet radiation.

<u>**Key causes of pre-mature aging**</u>

a. Heredity, health, sustainability, and psychosis. It can also be caused by stress and hormonal changes.
b. Free radicals—The prevention of free radicals which attack our cells. With a well balanced diet, rich in proteins, fruits and vegetables, vitamins and other relevant recommended diet, this will reduce the aging process.
c. Sunlight—Especially between 10 am to 3pm, always use sunscreen on the face and skin.
d. Lack of moisture. Use a good moisturizer.
e. Smoking
   This tends to accelerate the natural aging process of the skin, causing wrinkles. This can be caused by the contents of cigarettes which increases blood flow affect of the skin.
f. Excessive alcohol—You most reduce your intake.

<u>**Preventing pre-mature aging**</u>

1. Avoid the midday sun between the hours of 10 am to 4pm and use sunscreen every day. This can also give protection in disorders such as skin cancer. The use of lenses and shades, can block the ultra violet rays of the sun, and will protect the delicate skin around the eyes. You can also use umbrellas and hats.
2. Mind the way you sleep, because sleeping face down over the years, can cause sleep lines.

3. Avoid smoking, studies have shown that heavy smokers are five times more wrinkled than non-smokers. Tobacco tends to cause the acceleration of wrinkles by damaging the collagen layer and movement of the mouth when smoking tends to create wrinkles around the mouth area.

4. Use a good moisturizer for your skin; this will help the skin to retain moisture.

5. If you tend to frown a lot or come up with certain regular facial expressions, try to change that habit.

6. Avoid sun bathing and indoor tanning lamps and beds.

7. Eat well balanced diet and drink enough water daily.

8. Minimize on your alcohol intake.

9. Learn how to relax and ease you stress.

10. Exercise regularly.

**AVOID THE MIDDAY SUN BETWEEN
THE HOURS OF 10 A.M TO 4PM**

5.50   Age defying beauty secrets

People in their twenties

If you are in this age range, you will most likely have an oily skin and will most likely have occasional acne and pimples. After the age of 20, the amount of collagen which assists in keeping the skin plump and firm decreases by about one percent per year. During this stage, the appearance of wrinkles is low. The sun breaks down the collagen and seventy eight percent of sun damage is done usually before the age of 18 according to Arnold. W. Klein, MD at Beverly Hills' dermatologist clinic and professor at the University Of California School of medicine. According to him, the skin has the ability to repair itself, but you shouldn't keep insulting it. The most important thing is to use sunscreen judiciously.

What you can use

1. Use toners for oily skin.
2. Soaps and cleansers with benzoyl peroxide or salicylic acid for acne.
3. Oil free moisturizer only if necessary.
4. Broad spectrum sun screen with a sun protection factor of at least 15.

What a dermatologist can do for you

1. Treat acne and early signs of sun damage with glycolic acid peel (50% to 70% strength) Retin A or in extreme cases, acutance.

People in their thirties

At 30 aging tends to begin, your skin gets stiffer because you lose collagen and elastic fibers that are the key support structures. The skin also gets drier due to a slow decline in oil production. The skin tends to thin because you lose fat pads and it starts to sag from gravity pull. The skin also ages from the surface.

People at this age range are likely to have normal (that is combination) skin that is oily in the T-zone, adult acne from stress and pregnancy, birth control pills, fertility drugs, early signs of crow's feet, smile lines, forehead creases, frown lines, thinning lips.

What you can use

1. Gentle soap or cleanser.
2. Toner for normal skin.

3. Water base moisturizer.
4. Sun screen.
5. AHAS and other exfoliates.

What a dermatologist can do

Treat sun damage with retin A and glycolic acid peels (50% to 70% strength) to minimize pores, soften fine lines and improve skin tone.

For people in their forties

At this stage of life, people usually will expect normal skin with an increasingly dry T-one, crow's feet, smile lines from nose to month, forehead creases, frown lines, lines above lips especially if you smoke, underage bags, thinning lips, dilated pores on the nose from oil glands that enlarge with age, sun damage in the form of age spots, actinic keratoses. After forty the skin does not rejuvenate as quickly and as a result people should be careful about weight loss and gain.

What you can do

1. Use cleansing creams.
2. Toner.
3. AHAS and other exfoliates.
4. Water based moisturizer.
5. Eye cream and sun screen sun shades.

What a dermatologist can do

1. Treat sun damage with retin A or glycolic acid peels, acne or acne rosacea with retin A or acutance, sun spots and actinic keratoses with liquid nitrogen or a laser, use fillers (collagen, fat transplants, fibrel) or mild trichloroacetic acid peels to smooth out lines and plump up lips and botox to relax deep frown lines on the forehead.

For people in their fifties

At this stage of life, people will expect their skin to be drier, for women there can be adult acne that can flare up with menopause, the loss of elastic fibers in the skin increases considerably after the age of 50 and an eye lid drop is quite common, under eye bags, marionette lines (from corners of the mouth to chin), the tip of the nose begins to drop, the ears starts to elongate, and the jaw lines becomes less angular, because of underlying bone loss.

What you can do

1. Use oil based soaps and cleansers.
2. Alcohol-free toner.
3. Moisturizer.
4. AHAS and other exfoliates.
5. Eye cream.
6. Sun screen.
7. Sun shades.

What a dermatologist might do

I. Use fillers, tricholoroctetic acid peels etc

For people in their sixties

At this stage, the problems encountered when you were in your fifties will be very visible and the lower third of the face collapses because as we get older we lose our facial skeleton and at this stage most peoples chin will fall down and some are likely to lose their dentition.

What to do

1. Use soap and cleanser.
2. Use Alcohol-free toner.
3. Use oil based day moisturizer and night cream.
4. AHAS and other exfoliates.
5. Eye cream and sun screen.
6. Sun shades.

What a dermatologist can do

Use fillers, tricholorocteric acid peels etc

AT 30 AGING TENDS TO BEGIN

5.60   10 Ways to protect your heart

1. Lower your blood pressure which puts extra strain on your heart and arteries.
2. Get up on your backs, don't just wake up in the morning take your bath, watch television, sleep again, wake up and eat. This is dangerous, you must take a walk and do some exercise.
3. Reduce your alcohol intake or avoid it entirely. People who drink three or more alcoholic beverages a day are likely to develop high blood pressure and heavy drinkers can also develop cancer of the mouth, throat and liver.
4. Stop smoking, it raises blood pressure and increases heart disease. Smoking a stick of cigarette can raise blood pressure for up to I hour. Studies have shown that After I year smoke free, your heart disease risk will reduce by 50% and after 10-15 years smoke free, this risk is as low as one who never smoked before.
5. Reduce your weight in relationship to your height and heredity.
6. Know how to relax and manage your stress.
7. Reduce your intake of foods high in saturated fat such as beef, pork, eggs, butter, margarine, salad dressing etc.
8. Reduce your salt consumption.
9. Increase the intake of fruits and vegetables, whole grains and cereals, beans, peas etc.
10. Reduce your intake of refined and processed sugar and foods high sugar.

**A STICK OF CIGARATTE CAN RAISE
BLOOD PRESSURE FOR UP TO I HOUR**

5.70 Factors that cause breast cancer in women

1. Aging

   As women get older, they are at a higher risk of breast cancer. From 40 and above the risk tend to be higher and the risks are lower below this range.

2. Drinking more than the usual alcoholic limit. It is better not to drink more than one or two alcoholic beverages per day.

3. Deficiency in vitamin A, which can be found in carrots and other oranges and yellow vegetables.

4. Heredity

   People whose family members have suffered from breast cancer tend to have higher risk of this disorder and must try to avoid any form of life style or eating that can trigger it.

5. Excessive exposure to the sun radiation. You must use sunscreen between the hours when the suns radiation is at its peak, usually between 10 am and 4pm.

6. Excess body weight.

7. Not having biological children.

8. Smoking puts you at a higher risk.

9. Occasionally hormone replacement therapy can put you at risk.

10. Poor dieting.

    Not eating a balanced diet and eating a lot of high calories foods and low nutrient dense foods.

11. Lack of exercise.

12. Certain kinds of non cancerous breast cancer such as hyperplasia.

PEOPLE WHOSE FAMILY MEMBERS HAVE SUFFERED FROM BREAST CANCER TEND TO HAVE HIGHER RISK OF THIS DISORDER

5.80 11 Ways to avoid cancer in women

1. Stop smoking including other tobaccos.
2. Limit your intake of salt and nitrite cured foods.
3. Minimize on excess fat in your diet, particularly saturated fat.
4. Reduce on the calorie intake in your diet. Stick on the recommended limit for women.
5. Keep an eye on your weight
   Being overweight especially in post menopausal women can contribute to the risk of breast cancer and can further prevent its detection.

6. Exercise regularly because women who tend to exercise at least three hours per week in the early years of menstruation cut their risk of breast cancer by 30% from a number of studies.
7. Women should do their child bearing as early as possible, ideally before the age of 30 years.
8. Avoid other carcinogens like asbestos and other environmental pollutants.
9. Dermatologist and Oncologist tend to warn women to avoid excessive exposure to the sun light. In situation of inevitable exposure, it is necessary to use sunscreen for protection. Skin cancer has become more common due to the excessive exposure to the sun light.
10. Taking antioxidants in form of supplements can also offer some element of protection form cancer.
11. Consume diets that are rich in fruits, vegetables, beans and other high fiber foods. The foods most associated with cancer reduction usually contain antioxidants beta carotene, the plant form of vitamin A, and Vitamin C and E. People, who consume the greatest amount of antioxidants, tend to have a lower risk of all forms of cancers.

PEOPLE WHO CONSUME THE GREATEST AMOUNT OF ANTIOXIDANTS TEND TO HAVE A LOWER RISK OF ALL FORMS OF CANCERS

5.90   Early signs of breast cancer in women

1. Regular and persistence eczema in the form of rash in the nipple which seem to be unusual and you haven't had before.
2. You notice that your breast or breasts look or feel unusual and doesn't seem to go back to normal then see your doctor.
3. A change in the color of your nipple or obvious veins in your breast.
4. A change in the appearance of one or both nipples.
5. Discharge from the nipples particularly if the discharge is bloody and comes out without application of pressure.
6. Dimpling of the skin on your breast or breasts

Common tools for defecting breast cancer

1. Breast self exam.

    One method is called mamma care method. This is done by using your fingers to read and feel your breast by pressing your breast deep and deeper to get to the bottom your breast. To increase your chances of covering all the important breast tissue you must lie on your side and then twist slightly so that the breast that would normally hang down to your side is flattened across your chest and easier to palpate.

2. Visit your doctor for proper examination of your breast to know if you have a bad lump.

DISCHARGE FROM THE NIPPLES, PARTICULARLY IF THE DISCHARGE IS BLOODY AND COMES OUT WITHOUT APPLICATION OF PRESSURE TO YOUR BREAST

CHAPTER 6

6.00   Kidney disorder and Prevention

The kidney and urinary system maintain the chemical balance of all body fluids. The kidney filters out and removes waste products from the blood, maintains the normal level of nutrients in the blood and removes and excretes excess amounts of minerals, vitamins and other compounds. They also regulate the normal acid based (PH) balance in our body.

Some kidney disorders can be classed as acute and chronic kidney failure, kidney stones, nephorosis etc. Kidney stones seem to be common in diets high in protein, refined carbohydrates, fat, alcohol and phosphorus.

Prevention of kidney disorder

1. Try to consume a low fat high fiber nutrients dense foods adequate in all vitamin and minerals and low in sugar, refined and convenience foods.
2. Ensure you take several glasses of water daily in the region of 6-8 glasses.
3. Support your diet with some multiple vitamins and minerals supplement.
4. Cut down on the use of bubble baths and hygiene sprays.
5. Limit your intake of alcohol.
6. Avoid tobacco.
7. Coffee, tea and spicy foods is best avoided if you are infected.

> **THE KIDNEY FILTERS OUT AND REMOVES WASTE PRODUCTS FROM THE BLOOD**

6.10 Liver disorders and Prevention

The liver is the largest and one of the most important organs in our body and has a lot of function. Most of the nutrients absorbed from our diet are transported directly to the liver for storage, repackaging or combining with other compounds. Both the poisons that enter the body and the ones produced in the body are detoxified in the liver and it is very vital that our liver is functioning at its best.

Many compounds essential for growth and development are produced in the liver. In summary, the liver acts as a store house for nutrients. It converts vitamins to their active forms, such as carotene into vitamin A. Some of the diseases of the liver are hepatitis, cirrhosis, jaundice etc.

Prevention of liver disorders

1. Limit the intake of alcohol.
2. Avoid tobacco.
3. Consume low fat high fiber, nutrients dense diet.
4. Cut down on the intake of sugar, refined and convenience foods.
5. Support your diet with a daily intake of nutrients and minerals supplements.
6. Drink adequate water daily 6-8 glasses.
7. Consume fresh juice such as apples, oranges, pineapples, carrots, cranberries and vegetables daily.
8. Maintain regular exercise and learn to relax and manage stress.

POISONS THAT ENTERS THE BODY AND THE ONES PRODUCED IN THE BODY ARE DETOXIFIED IN THE LIVER

6.20   Typhoid fever and Prevention

Typhoid fever is caused by a small bacterium called salmonella typhi. Typhoid tends to be very common in dirty environment and can be contracted through contaminated foods, drinks, house flies etc.

The common symptoms of typhoid are headache, fever, pains, weakness, vomiting, loss of appetite, bitterness of the mouth and internal heat etc.

Prevention of typhoid disorder

1. Ensure that your foods are not exposed to house flies.
2. Wash vegetables, fruits and other edibles, thoroughly with water before intake.
3. Ensure that you don't consume foods left uncovered.
4. Ensure that your foods are heated properly, do not form the habit of eating cold foods.
5. Ensure that your drinking water is treated properly.
6. Ensure that you don't eat expired foods.

```
TYPHOID TENDS TO BE VERY
COMMON IN DIRTY
ENVIRONMENTS
```

6.30   Arthritis disorder and Prevention

Arthritis is classed as the inflammation of the joint. It is an autoimmune disease, a condition affecting the skin and other vital organs. The common feature of these disorders such as rheumatoid gouty and osteoarthritis is an odd sensitivity of the immune system, one that causes it to attack the body's own tissues as unwelcomed foreign substances.

The symptoms of rheumatoid arthritis vary with the stage of the disorder. At the first stage, those affected tend to complain of fatigue and feeling sore, achy, and stiffening of joints. The cause of rheumatoid arthritis seems to be unclear and is possibly a combination of a disturbance in the body's immune response, infection, heredity and many other factors.

Osteoarthritis is the most popular form of arthritis found in older people. It is a degeneration of the cartilage of the joints of the knees, feet, toes, hips, ankles, and backbone. This cause can be as a result of physical stress experienced throughout life, injuries, other joint diseases and obesity.

Joint pain and stiffness tend to be more pronounced when the patient is malnourished and deficiencies of folic acid, vitamin C, vitamin D, Vitamin B4, vitamin B12, iron, Magnesium and Zinc.

Arthritis Prevention

1. Ensure that you add several antioxidants nutrients to your diet. Such as vitamin C in the range of orange juice, tomatoes, strawberries, cabbage, green peas, carrots, pineapple etc. Vitamin E range such as wheat germs, nuts, avocado, Beta-carotene, the plant form of vitamin A such as Dark green, apple, garden egg, lettuce, melon, sweet potatoes etc.
Selenium such as grains, lean meat, organ meat and fish.

2. Fish oils—The fatty acid found in fish oil can be useful for this ailment. People, who took fish capsules, have reported improvement in morning stiffness.
3. A low fat high fiber nutrients dense foods low in sugar and refined and convenience foods are always helpful.
4. Undertake regular exercise and manage your stress.
5. Avoid alcohol and tobacco.

6. Regular massage and heat can reduce the pain of rheumatoid arthritis.

OSTEOARTHRITIS IS THE MOST POPULAR FORM OF ARTHRITIS FOUND IN MAJORITY OF OLDER PEOPLE

6.40 Asthma and Prevention

Asthma is one of the most common health problems. It is a condition where the patients have repeated attacks of wheezing which usually clears up completely with medication. Attacks produce a variety of disabilities from mild distress to severe one. Asthma can develop anytime in life, but usually starts at childhood.

Wheezing a lot is one of the symptoms of asthma, cough sometimes accompanies it, pulse rate raises and inability to speak due to breathlessness. There is also typical difficulty in breathing out rather than breathing in.

Causes

In asthmatic patients, the bronchial tube muscles, which transport air to the air spaces in the lungs, become narrow due to contraction, and air cannot move freely in or out of the lungs. Bronchial tubes also produce more mucous than usual which further reduces air movement.

Certain drugs a patient is allergic to can trigger an asthma attack including emotional trauma, anger, sudden fluctuation in weather or temperature etc. In reality the causes of asthma are unclear and can also result from heredity, food allergies etc.

Asthma prevention

1. Increase in the intake of vitamin B6 which can reduce the symptoms; however your doctor must be the focal point of this supervision.
2. A strict vegetarian or vegan diet and avoidance of all foods in animal origin are necessary.
3. Avoid alcohol and tobacco.
4. Avoid food additives such as flavor enhancers, coloring agent and preservatives.
5. Ensure you undertake regular exercise and manage your stress.
6. Avoid all cold foods such as ice cream, yogurt, milk, cold cucumber, cold drinks and lemon etc.

7. Take note of your Allergies, triggering foods or medications.

> **IN ASTHMATIC PATIENTS, THE BRONCHIAL TUBE MUSCLES WHICH TREANSPORTS AIR TO THE AIR SPACES IN THE LUNGS BECOME NARROW**

6.50   Tooth disorder and Prevention

Good teeth is an indication of good health, but often these are prone to infections because they are exposed to a varieties of foods and drinks and tooth ache appear to be the most popular complaint.

Causes

The main cause of tooth ache is the decay of the teeth, resulting from bad eating habits such as over indulgence in sweets, ice creams, soft drinks, and sugary foods.

Bacteria present in the mouth cavity break sugar down into acids, which interact with the calcium in the enamel to cause decay or erosion.

Signs and Symptoms

Tooth ache may be constant throughout the day and night or it may come and go occasionally depending on the degree of decay. The character of the pain may be dull, sharp, shooting or radiating towards the ears and head, severe headaches can follow.

Toothache disorder prevention

1. Limit your intake of sugary foods such as jams, jellies desserts, candies, heavily sugared beverages, soft drinks, sweets and sugary biscuits etc.
2. Consumption of raw and rough foods such as carrots, apples, green salads, scrape the teeth and help to prevent accumulation of plague and the development of tooth decay.
3. Nursing mothers should not expose their infants to nursing bottle syndrome. This is a condition in infants and small children characterized by extensive decay and loss of upper teeth. They can be prevented by not giving the child a bottle at bedtime filled with any beverage that contains sugar, sugared fruits, orange juice, instead give the child water.
4. Daily use of fluoride tooth paste and mouth wash twice daily will go a long way to keep your teeth healthy.

5. You must brush your teeth in the morning and in the night before bedtime.

> **BACTERIA PRESENT IN THE MOUTH CAVITY BREAK SUGAR DOWN INTO ACIDS WHICH INTERACT WITH THE CALCIUM IN THE ENAMEL TO CAUSE DECAY**

6.60   Eye disorders and Prevention

A good eye sight is an indication of a healthy eye, while the reverse is the case for a poor eye sight. Generally as we get older our eye sight tend to reduce.

The most common eye problem that cuts across all age groups is short sight (myopia) and long sight. Short sight refers to difficulty in seeing objects at a distance. Long sight is the reverse. Myopia seems to be more common and can be due to the change in the curvature of the refracting surface of the eye or abnormal refractivity of the media of the eye. Myopia can be as a result of prolonged viewing of television, working with computers etc.

Another common eye problem that seems to be very common with older people is called cataract. Pacification of the lens of the eye or its covering, sufficient to interfere with vision is called cataract.

Causes

Malnutrition, deficiencies in vitamin A or B, high myopia (short sight), diabetes, old age, infection of the eye etc.

Signs and symptoms

Initially patient complains of blurring vision in the early stays of the disorder. When the cataract matures, complete vision is lost in the affected eye. If treatment is not undertaken, the cataract becomes hyper mature and can lead to increase in intra-ocular pressure (Glaucoma).

Eye disorder preventions

1. Ensure that your diet is not deficient in fish oil. The Omega 3 fatty acids in fish oil are very good for a good eye sight.
2. Your diet must contain the recommended proportion of vitamin A, which is necessary for the development and manufacture of normal eye tissue and vision. A condition known as night blindness is an early sign of deficiency in vitamin A. A person suffering from night blindness seems to struggle in seeing in deem light. And if the deficiently in vitamin A continues, it can lead to irreversible loss of vision. Some symptoms of vitamin A deficiency include over sensitivity to bright lights, itching or burning sensation in the eye, dryness of eyelids etc. To reverse

these damages, you should increase your intake of vitamin A and vitamin A rich foods such as dark green vegetables, fruits such as apple, carrots etc.

3. Vitamin E as an antioxidant protects the eyes from damage caused by highly reactive compounds known as free radicals discussed earlier. It helps to prevent several eye disorders including cataract formation. Some of the sources of vitamin E in our diet are vegetable oils, seeds, wheat germs, and nuts.

4. Deficiency in vitamin B2 can lead to damage to the eye tissue, poor vision, burning and itching in the eyes and increased blood vessels in the eye. Increase in the intake of vitamin B2 rich foods is very important to prevent this disorder. Some of the vitamin B2 rich foods are milk and low fat daily products, dark green leafy vegetables etc.

5. Vitamin C can inhibit the progression and encourage the regression of some forms of cataract. Vitamin C rich diets are oranges, tomatoes, carrots, cabbage, strawberries, potato, melon and pineapples etc.

VITAMIN E AS AN ANTIOXIDANT PROTECTS THE EYES FROM DAMAGE CAUSED BY HIGHLY REACTIVE COMPOUNDS KNOWN AS FREE RADICALS

6.70 Anemia

In reality anemia means "without blood". It is a reduction in the number or size of red blood cells or the amount of hemoglobin within the cells. There are many types of anemia, however iron deficiency accounts for a considerable proportion of the disorder.

Causes

1. Bleeding such as heavy periods in women appears to be the main cause in women. The condition can also be as a result of excessive destruction of red blood cells and the bone marrow cannot produce enough to replace those that are damaged.
2. Dietary deficiency of iron, vitamin B12, folic acid, vitamin B6, vitamin C and E.
3. Insufficient production of Red Blood Cells (RBC) due to a number of factors, such as iron deficiency anemia, vitamin deficiency anemia and pernicious anemia are both forms of anemia in which there are inadequate supply of vitamin B12 and folic acids.

Signs and symptoms

1. Feeling of tiredness because the body is not getting enough oxygen.
2. Loss of the healthy gloom of the skin and the face looking pale.
3. In severe circumstances of anemia the person will experience short of breath and the ankle may swell.

Anemia prevention

1. Eat iron rich foods from animal's sources such as liver, tongue, heart and other organ meat, lean meat, fish and eggs.
2. Enjoy several servings of fresh fruits and vegetables, whole grains and milk products.
3. Take a daily vitamin supplement containing iron, vitamin B12, B6, folic acid, vitamin C, vitamin E and copper.
4. Sleep at least 8 hours at night.

> **IN SEVERE CIRCUMSTANCES OF ANEMIA THE PERSON WILL EXPERIENCE SHORT OF BREATH AND THE ANKLE MAY SWELL**

6.80 Lung disorder and Prevention

The lungs key role is to supply the blood stream with oxygen and remove unwanted gases such as carbon dioxide, from the system. Carton dioxide is removed with each exhalation and oxygen absorbed into the blood stream with each inhalation.

This exchange of gases is called respiration. Our lungs are exposed to many environmental substances that can cause infections, such as molds, bacteria, viruses, pollens etc. However the enzymes in our respiratory track tend to destroy foreign substances inhaled into the lungs. The epithelial linings that forms a physical barrier to contaminants, the mucous coating that covers the epithelial lining of the lungs, also prevents the invasion by harmful germs and substances and a layer of minute hair like structures (Cilia) on the lining of the respiratory track sweep inhaled debris into the stomach for excretion. This protects the lungs from inhaled germs.

Tobacco inhalation, alcohol, and air pollutions, weakens the lining of the lungs and reduces the strength of the immune system which subsequently increases our lungs chances of contracting diseases and infections.

Some of the common lungs disorders are bronchitis, emphysema, lung cancer etc.

Lung disorders and prevention

1. Maintain a healthy immune system, combined with an active antioxidant system. Consume a low fat, high fiber nutrient dense diet which is adequate in all vitamins and minerals and low in sugar, refined and convenience foods.
2. Avoid tobacco use and being around people that tend to smoke.
3. Limit your exposure to air pollution and other toxic gases.
4. Limit your intake of alcohol.
5. Undertake regular exercise and manage you stress.
6. Ensure a reasonable daily consumption of fruits such as apples, carrots, melon, orange, pawpaw, and vegetables.

> **TOBACCO INHALATION, ALCOHOL AND AIR POLLUTION WEAKENS THE LINING OF THE LUNGS**

6.90   Malaria fever and Prevention

Malaria is a common fever that is prevalent in tropical regions such as Africa, India etc. Malaria fever is caused by plasmodium, a single celled organism that thrives in the red blood cells of its victims. The plasmodium parasite is spread from one person to another through mosquito bites. When the mosquito sucks the blood of the infected person, it spreads it to another person through a bite. The most dangerous member of the plasmodium family is plasmodium falciparum.

Signs and symptoms

1. Flulike symptoms, including a severe headache, body aches and pains in the muscles and joints internal heat.
2. Shivering and high temperature. Temperature rise is dramatic and vomiting may occur. This is followed by a phase of heavy sweating and a fall in temperature. The circle of fever may come and go.

Malaria and prevention

1. Ensure that your body is not exposed to mosquito bite.
2. Ensure your environment is clean.
3. Use mosquito nets on doors and windows.
4. Ensure that old cans, broken bottles, and other related materials that breed mosquitoes are kept out of your house.
5. Improve your immune system by eating a balanced diet.
6. Limit the way you eat greasy foods and fats.
7. Increase your consumption of fruits and vegetables.

> **THE PLASMODIUM PARASITE IS SPREAD FROM ONE PERSON TO ANOTHER THROUGH MOSQUITO BITES**

6.100 <u>Acquired immune deficiency syndrome/prevention</u>

Acquired immune deficiency syndrome (Aids) is a progressive decease starting with HIV infection. It is characterized by the gradual suppression of the immune system during the HIV stage which subsequently leads to Aids. The suppression of the body's immune response means that the body's natural defense system against diseases and infections is seriously weakened, living the person to be open to easy infections.

The person usually does not die of Aids but from secondary infection such as cancer, tuberculosis, pneumonia etc.

<u>Diet and prevention</u>

1. HIV/Aids patients must concentrate on diets that help to build up the immune system (Refer to chapter 4 paragraph 4.70 and 4.80.
   a. Cut down on total fat consumption.
   b. Eat more high fiber foods such as whole grains, cereals, fruits and vegetables.
   c. Consume adequate amount of nutrients dense foods adequate in all vitamins and mineral and low in sugar, refined and convenience foods.
   d. Calorie intake should be adequate enough to maintain a normal body weight.
   e. A multiple vitamin mineral supplement that supplies at least 100% recommended dietary allowance should be consumed daily.
   f. Avoid tobacco and alcohol.
   g. Manage your stress.

2. Avoid pre-marital sex.
3. Know the status of your partner.
4. Use protection during sex i.e. condom.
5. Avoid blood contact with the infected person.
6. Avoid unscreened blood transfusion.

> **HIV/AIDS PATIENTS MUST CONCENTRATE ON DIETS THAT HELP TO BUILD UP THE IMMUNE SYSTEM**

6.110 <u>Gall bladder disorder and Prevention</u>

The causes of gall bladder remain debatable, some experts doubt that any one factor can be blamed and believes it is the sum total of several factors such as

1. Heredity—It tends to run in families.
2. Infection—This accounts for some cases.
3. Bile consumption—The main function of the gall bladder is to store bile, a substance needed in the digestive process. The factors which increase the cholesterol content of the bile are considered a strong factor on the health of the gall bladder. In United States around 20% of men and women tend to have gall stones.

Also growing older accounts for a higher risk of gall bladder disease and overweight, diabetes etc can put you at risk of gall bladder disease.

<u>Gall bladder disorder and Prevention.</u>

1. Reduce your calorie consumption. Over storage of calorie can be dangerous. The sources of calories are protein, carbohydrate, alcohol etc.
2. The Australian scientist R. K. R Scragg in his studies found that the chances of developing gall stones are increased if you tend to consume a lot of fat.
3. Eat more fiber from fruits and vegetables, British researcher K.W Keaton and his colleagues in their studies, found that a low fiber intake affects the bile consumption in a way that probably favor the development of gallstone.
4. Reduce your sugar consumption; people who consume large amount of sugar are extremely prone to gallstone.

> **THE CHANCES OF DEVELOPING GALL STONES IS INCREASED IF WE TEND TO CONSUME A LOT OF FAT**

6.120 Thyroid disorder and Prevention

The most common symptom of thyroid malfunctioning is enlargement of thyroid gland or goiter. The thyroid gland enlarges in an attempt to maintain normal function when there is an insufficient supply of iodine necessary for thyroxin production.

Poor dietary intake of iodine results in goiter in adults and if the diet is low in iodine during pregnancy, the baby will be born with a condition called cretinism. The function of iodine is as a component of thyroid hormones. Thyroid hormones regulate the rate of metabolism, growth, reproduction, nerve and muscle function, and the synthesis of proteins, the growth of the skin and hair, and the use of oxygen by cells.

One of the hormones called thyroxin regulates the rate at which the body uses energy from food and this is an important regulator of body weight. When the thyroid lacks iodine, the pituitary gland which is the main gland signals to the thyroid gland to increase its activity and these results to the swelling or enlargement of the thyroid gland, called goiter. Some foods contain goitrogens which are natural inhibitors of thyroid gland. Some of these foods are raw cabbage, peanuts, mustard seeds, cauliflower, soybeans and cassava. Too much intake of these foods when the diet is low in iodine can produce goiter.

Thyroid disorder prevention

1. Enhance your iodine, level, by consuming foods such as fresh water shell fish, sea foods, iodized salt etc.
2. You can also consider iodine supplements.

SOME FOODS CONTAIN GOISTROGENS WHICH ARE NATURAL INHIBITORS OF THYROID GLAND

CHAPTER 7

7.00 Infertility in women and men

Infertility in women

Infertility in women can be defined as the failure to achieve pregnancy after a one full year of unprotected intercourse or sex. If you cannot conceive for some years of unprotected sex, it does not mean that you are barren; however medical attention will be required in order to reverse most situations. There are some factors that can lead to women infertility.

1. It may be that your fecundity is low, that is your chances of becoming pregnant in any given month or menstrual cycle. For average fertile women, the fecundity rate is about 20% that is they have a one in five chance of becoming pregnant in every given cycle. These set of women are usually in their early to mid twenties. About 93% of these fecund women will usually become pregnant within one year while 50% will become pregnant just after 3 months. Age and other factors tend to reduce the fecundity rate of women.

2. There are considerable varieties of causes of infertility. For instance for conception to take place, a vast array of organ systems, hormonal signals, and other physical factors must be in place for both male and female. For instance the male sperm must be produced, and must be healthy, and must be able to travel out of a man's body and into the women.

3. There can be ovulation problems for instance an inability to create and release mature eggs which can occur any where along the brain reproductive organ path way.

4. The problem with the physical structures such as structural defect in the uterus, malfunctioning ovaries or blocked fallopian tubes.

5. Problem involving the health of the cervix, the mouth of the uterus which may produce less than ideal mucus, which tend to help usher the sperm into the uterus and into the tubes.

There were periods when the issue of infertility was thought to be caused by women alone, but those days are long gone. Dr Kaylen Silverberry, a reproductive endocrinologist at the University of Texas, San Antonio, says infertility is a team sports, couples should be treated for infertility not individually. It is thought that approximately 40% of infertility has some significant male factor, 40% has some significant female factor and about 20% involves both sexes.

In most cities, large percentage of infertility problems is caused by sexually transmitted diseases. Also Dr Michael Diamond of the Vanderbilt school of medicine, in his studies noticed that an increase in infertility in women was caused by delay in child bearing.

Infertility in men

In men there are different kinds of sperm problems and they are treated differently. Usually the sperm is studied for several characteristics which are usually the number of sperm on the semen, secondly the mobility of the sperm, that is how well they move and swim, thirdly morphology of the sperm, that is how the sperm is shaped, and fourthly the ability of the sperm to penetrate a test egg. Other infertility problems in men are blocked sperm, diet and not being able to produce a live sperm.

Fertility Foods for Men

a. Oysters

They have a considerable level of zinc. Oysters helps increase the production of sperm and testosterone like baby making ingredient. If you can't cope with this seafood, you can find zinc in food such as beef, poultry, dairy, nuts, eggs, whole grains and beans.

b. Fruits and Vegetables

The antioxidants found in fruits and vegetables such as dried fruits, cranberry, collard green, help protect the sperm from cellular damage and keep them strong and speedy. Just what they need to race through the fallopian tube and fertilize the egg.

Take vitamin A, which is important in preventing slow sperm.
Take vitamin C, which is critical for the sperm mobility and viability; consider tomatoes, orange juice, grape fruit, broccoli etc.

Take vitamin E, which helps keep sperm vibrant, consider vegetable oil, leafy greens, beans etc.

Also vitamin B, with antioxidant properties is crucial for keeping the sperm free of chromosol abnormalities.

One power food that is packed with all the nutrients above, vitamin A, C, E, and the folate is sweet potato. Other important diets are pomegranate juice, which tends to boost sperm count and quality, Pumpkin seeds, which contains a high dose of zinc, which increase testosterone and sperm count. They are also loaded with Omega fatty acids which stimulate blood flow to sexual organs and improve sexual function.

c. Garlic

Occasional dose of garlic can seriously improve your fertility.

d. Brazil nuts

Rich sources of selenium. Improves sperm count, it is known to increase the number of active sperm in the body while developing their mobility.

e. Oily fish with its essential fatty acids (EFAs)

Such as salmon, mackerel, sardine, improves blood circulation around the reproductive system and in the process boosts sperm quality.

f. Chili Pepper

Speed up the flow of blood to key reproductive areas.

Baby busting foods for men

1. Junk foods, such as doughnuts, French fries, hamburger etc.
2. High mercury fish, such as sword fish, king mackerel, tile fish etc.
3. Caffeinated drinks and alcohol, such as too much coffee, tea and alcohol.

Fertile foods for women

1. Red meat

Iron packed red meat can seriously lower the risk of infertility arising in the ovulating process. Iron helps to boost red blood cells while reducing the treat posed by anemia. Red meat also offers a good source of zinc, supporting ovulation and maintaining efficient cell division.

2. Nuts

   Nuts such as walnuts, almonds are high in vitamin E contents and increase the female sex drive, while simultaneously protecting embryos from miscarriages.

3. Oysters

   Oysters offer a good level of zinc which can prove vital to healthy ovulation and steady egg production. Alternatives can be found in eggs, beans and nuts etc.

4. Baked Potatoes

   They are high in vitamin B, which is perfect for vibrant love making. The contents in vitamin B and E found in these foods also enhance cell division; increase the chances of healthy Ova being produced.

Improving the Chances of the sex of a child

The males are the sole parties responsible for planning on the genetic codes to determine if a child will be a male or female.

It is quite obvious in biology that XX combination of sperm and egg creates a female, while the XY combination creates a male.

All eggs are X and sperm can be either X or Y. We must remember that the conception in the fallopian tube is the first sperm to reach and penetrate the surface of the egg. This conception is the result of a race amongst millions of little swimming sperms to reach the single available egg. (A small percentage of women ovulation on both sides simultaneously and has higher chances to create fraternal twins).

There are two kinds of sperm

1. The endosperm or male-genetic-code version.
2. The genosperm or the female.

Determining the sex of your child has to do with taking advantage of the unique characteristic of each. For simplicity let's call the boy "Toni" and the girl "Chelsea".

The endosperm or the male (Toni's) are smaller and swim faster, but they do not swim as far and do not last very long. Consider them the sprinters.

The genosperm or the female (Chelsea) are bigger and slower. They can last up to 36 hours in some vaginal environments. Consider them the long distance runners.

Men tend to increase the ratio of Toni's to Chelsea's in the load when there has been an extended period of lack of sex. This has been shown over the years where the first generation of children after men have been away at war has a higher proportion of males. Also certain cultures, who only engage in sexual intercourse once a month at the expected time of fertility, have a very high proportion of males in the range of 60% and above.

Chelsea's favor more acidic environments and Toni's like the basic.

There are five things to remember.

1. Penetration

The closer the point at which the load (the ejaculation) is delivered to the egg, the more likely a sprinter like the Toni's will win the race. Therefore for a better chance of a boy, stick it all the way inside when you reach climax.

2. Timing

If the load is delivered before the egg is available, the Toni's will die off and the Chelsea's will be there waiting. Ovulation usually takes place around the 14th day of the cycle, measured as day one, being the start of the menstrual period. Intercourse on the the 12th or 13th day will favor Chelsea because there will be no egg to fertilize for a day or two.

3. Viscosity

Vaginal liquids are relatively thick and present an impediment to the Chelsea's while Toni's swim right through this thick liquids.

To make boys, make her real happy (several times) prior to delivering the load. Try stimulating her properly before delivering the load.

4. Abstinence

If you do it every day, you will probably make a girl because the Toni's/Chelsea ratio in the ejaculate will decline. Therefore save it up a little if you want to improve your chances of a boy.

5. Acid/Base

Some couples use the acid containing vinegar to increase their chances of making girls and hence baking soda to improve their chances of making boys.

> **FOR AVERAGE FERTILE WOMEN,
> THE FECUNDITY RATE IS ABOUT
> 20%**

7.10 The important qualities of water

1. Water tends to work in the body's awareness resistance to diseases and increasing energy. Because we are warm blooded, we tend to react very sensitively to changes in temperature. These reactions activate all the important body systems and stabilize the body and increase the use of oxygen in the cells. Warm water dilates blood vessels, thus improving blood circulation, which improve the flow of oxygen to the brain and fasten the elimination of toxins from our body. Hydrotherapy will not only achieve a well balanced body but also a healthy mind.

2. The body of an adult consists of about 60% water; it is a part of every body cell. Children above 5 years of age may have about 70% water and children under 5 years of age may have about 75% water. Children need to drink even more water than adults.

3. Our kidney filters about 1,600 liters of blood every day (400 gallons), yet only about one and half liters of urine is voided in a day. One half of a liter (2 glassful of water) is lost in a day through the breath and about the same amount or much more in hot climates in lost through invisible or visible perspiration. Through the bowels about one third of a liter is lost in a stool. Therefore the average loss of water in a day from an adult's body is about two and half liters to three liters or more (10 glasses or more). The more glass of water we drink to replace this lost water, the better for our body and the less we dehydrate.

4. A lot of people suffer from constipation because they do not drink enough water to keep the stool soft. Lack of fiber can also cause this.

5. The best habit to form during your life is to drink at least two glasses of water when you get out of bed in the morning. The balance of the body's daily need for water should ideally be taken into the body 30 minutes before meals or two and half hours after meals. This practice encourages better digestion. To drink a lot of fluids at meals time is not good physiologically and tends to slow down digestion.

6. For diabetic, stroke, ulcer patients, drinking enough water, coupled with the recommended doctor's medication will go a long way in improving health.

> **A LOT OF PEOPLE SUFFER FROM CONSTIPATION BECAUSE THEY DO NOT DRINK ENOUGH WATER**

7.20 Vitamins that give longevity and keep you younger

Vitamins are necessary for life. Vitamin with the help of minerals maintains the proper functioning of the body and regulate metabolism. Some key vitamins that will help us live longer and look younger are,

Fat Soluble

1a. Fat soluble

Vitamin A, D, E and K, require the fat carriers to be absorbed and not as easily assimilated as water soluble vitamins. Fat free foods interfere with these vitamins since fatty acids are needed for their absorption.

1b. Water soluble

Vitamin C, bioflavoid, and vitamin B including choline, and inositol are easier to assimilate because they dissolve in water, since vitamins are eliminated through the urine; they need to be replenished more often than fat soluble vitamins.

2 Vitamin A, and Beta carotene
   a. They assist the body to fight and prevent infections.
   b. Helps the body to remove waste.
   c. Protect the body from free radicals.
   d. Very important for pregnancy.
   e. Keeps the reproductive organ in good health.
   f. Encourages healthy skin, teeth, bone, hair etc.
   g. Promotes good vision.

These vitamins are available in spinach, carrots, green leaves, spirulina etc.

3 Vitamin B1 (Thiamine) Borale vitamin.
   a. Helps in stressful times.
   b. Necessary for the development of muscle.
   c. Necessary for growth.
   d. Necessary for digestion and absorption of nutrients.
   e. Keeps the heart in good health.
   f. Promotes the metabolism of carbohydrates.

These vitamins are available in fish, peanuts, spirulina etc.

4 Vitamin B2 (Riboflavin)
   a. Very necessary for reproduction.

123

    b. Promotes growth, healthy skin, nail, hands and digestive system.

These vitamins are available in grains, spirulua etc.

5 Vitamin B3 (Niacin)
    a. Assists in digestion.
    b. Promotes healthy skin.
    c. Helps in insulin production.
    d. Promotes healthy sperm and ovaries.
    e. Promotes good circulation.
    f. Helps to eliminate bad cholesterol.

These vitamins are available in milk, peanut, spirulina, chickens breast etc.

6 Niacinamide or Nicotinamide
    a. Helps in digestion.
    b. Helps in the treatment of diabetes.
    c. Helps in the treatment of rheumatoid and osteo-arthritis.
    d. Helps in cholesterol reduction.

This vitamin can be found in spirulina.

7 Vitamin B5 (Pantothenic acid)
    a. Helps to convert food to energy.
    b. Assists the body in fighting diseases.
    c. Helps the gland to function well.
    d. Helps to prevent stress.
    e. Promotes the healing of injury.
    f. Promotes growth.
    g. Promotes long life.

These vitamins is found in spirulina, Grains, orange etc

8 Vitamin B6 (Pyridoxine)
    a. Necessary for protein metabolism.
    b. Necessary for the absorption of vitamin B12.
    c. Necessary for cell formation.
    d. Helps fatty acids to function properly.
    e. Necessary for healthy muscles, nerves, skin and teeth.
    f. Promotes the health of the liver.

9   Vitamin B12 (Cobalamin)
   a. Helps in anemia and fatigue.
   b. Helps in cell formation.
   c. Helps in energy production.
   d. Assists other vitamins to function properly.
   e. Helps to improve the brain.
   f. Improves circulation.
   g. Promotes growth and healthy nerves.

This vitamin can be found in spirulina, fish, egg, milk etc.

10 Biotin
   a. Helps in the metabolism of fats and carbohydrates.
   b. Helps in the formation of cells.
   c. Helps other vitamin B, to function properly.
   d. Prevents loss of hair.
   e. Helps reduce stress.

This vitamin can be found in eggs, Grains, soy, spirulina etc.

11 Folic Acid
   a. Helps vitamin B12 to produce healthy red blood cells.
   b. Prevents and treats anemia.
   c. Important for normal fetal development.
   d. Necessary during pregnancy.
   e. Necessary for proper functioning of the brain and neurotransmitter.
   f. Work with vitamin C and B12 for the body to use protein.
   g. Stimulates appetite and stomach acid and support the liver to work properly.
   h. Works well with vitamin C, E and B.
   Folic acid can be found in milk, spirulina, spinach, green leaves etc.

12 Vitamin C
   a. Helps fight infections.
   b. Helps to maintain protein collagen.
   c. Strengthens body tissues.
   d. Appears to be the best antioxidants.
   e. Protects the body from damage from free radicals.
   f. Prevents premature aging.

g. High dose prevents and destroys candida bacteria and degenerative ailments.

h. Assists in healing injury.

i. Repairs cells and reduces bad cholesterol.

This vitamin can be found in tomatoes, oranges, spirulina etc.

13 Vitamin E

a. A strong antioxidant.

b. Protects the body from pollution, toxins and free radicals.

c. Prevents premature aging, cancer, impotence, heart and degenerative diseases.

d. Heals injury and prevents scarring.

e. Prevents miscarriage.

f. Prevents blood clots and reduces bad cholesterol.

g. Enhances the action of vitamin A, C, and fatty acids.

This vitamin can be found in spirulina, egg, vegetable oils, tomatoes etc.

14 Vitamin K

a. Helps to maintain healthy blood clotting.

b. Prevents life threatening blood bleeding.

c. Needed to store carbohydrates and supports bone structure.

d. Helps to prolong life, important key to longevity.

e. Helps the liver to function normal.

This vitamin can be found in spirulina, plant chlorophyll etc.

15 Calcium

a. Forms and maintain strong bones and teeth.

b. Helps for normal muscle contraction.

c. Prevents osteoporosis.

d. Depends upon vitamin A,C and D for good absorption.

e. Works best with magnesium.

f. Maintains the cardiovascular system.

This vitamin can be found in milk, spirulina, almonds etc.

16 Magnesium

a. Works with calcium and phosphorus.

b. Build bones, conducts nerve impulses and contracts muscles.

    c. Increases enzyme activity during metabolism for the production of energy in the brain, heart and organs of the body.

    d. Magnesium helps to avoid the heart and blood vessels problem.

    e. Work with vitamin B6 to cause enzymatic reaction.

    f. Helps to convert sugar in the blood into energy.

This vitamin can be found in garlic, onion, almond, spirulina, Gura, lime, etc.

17 Phosphorus

    a. Helps calcium for nerve conduction and muscle contraction.

    b. Works with calcium to improve the bone structure and teeth.

    c. Promotes good functioning of the brain.

This vitamin can be found in milk, fish, grain, egg, spirulina, etc.

18 Iron

    a. Helps in the transportation of oxygen in red blood cells.

    b. Prevents anemia.

    c. Involves in body functions, enzymatic reactions, and necessary for energy, metabolism and DNA.

    d. Treats and prevents blood loss.

This vitamin can be found in fish, egg, spirulina, green leaves, yam back, plantain etc.

19 Zinc

    a. Helps the immune system to fight infection.

    b. Improves the health of the skin.

    c. Helps the wound to heal faster.

    d. Necessary for the production of many hormones.

    e. Supports healthy reproductive system.

    f. Used for the prevention and treatment of prostrate problems.

    g. Increases sense of smell, taste and vision.

    h. Assists the body to produce insulin.

    i. Boosts healthy sperm production.

This vitamin can be found in mushrooms, sunflower products, spirulina etc.

20 Selenium

    a. An antioxidant which works with vitamin E.

    b. Prevents aging.

    c. Prevents cancer and heart disease.

    d. Promotes growth and fertility.

e. Necessary for the production of prostaglandins.

f. Needed for the utilization of essential fatty acids and treats inflammation.

This vitamin can be found in grains, spirulina, rice, meats.

21 Silicon

a. Helps firm the skin and improves its elasticity.

b. Helps to harden nails and promotes thick hair.

c. Strengthens bones structure and connective tissues.

d. Prevents arteriosclerosis and heart disease.

e. Helps to prolong life by preventing the cells from aging.

This vitamin can be found in lettuce, almonds, spirulina, spinach etc.

> **MAGNESSIUM HELP TO PREVENT HEART AND BLOOD VESSELS PROBLEMS**

7.30 Preventing hypertension (High Blood Pressure)

Hypertension refers to an increase in the blood pressure of an individual. Blood pressure is the blood force against the wall of the arteries and the heart as the blood is pumped from the heart to the tissues. Therefore hypertension is blood pressure that remains above the normal range and indicates a steady excessive pumping of blood against the walls of the arteries and heart. Hypertension is one of the three primary risk factors for the development of cardiovascular disease, heart attack, and stroke. The best defense against hypertension is to prevent it and the second best defense is to control the existing hypertension with diet, life style, habits, exercise and medication.

Causes

In more than 95% of cases, no special cause can be found and such patients are said to have essential hypertension and in most circumstances when we go to the doctors surgery we are usually tense and nervous, which tends to increase our blood pressure, this is called white coat hypertension, however this tends to settle as we become more relaxed. However if the blood pressure registers a steady level above the normal range over a period of time and taken over different time of the day, this is usually an issue of concern and require the attention of a doctor.

In some cases hypertension may be secondary to some diseases or abnormality leading to secondary hypertension. Some of the causes of hypertension are

1. Excessive alcohol intake.
2. Excessive salt intake.
3. Lack of exercise.
4. Being over weight.
5. Heredity.
6. Stress and mental tension.
7. Poor diets, usually diets high in saturated fat.
8. Pregnancy.
9. Disease of the kidney.
10. Hormonal disorders.
11. Certain drugs such as contraceptive pills, pain killers etc.
12. Smoking.

Signs and symptoms

Headache, dizziness, palpitation, lack of sleep, breathlessness on exertion, easy fatigability etc.

Prevention

1. Maintenance of an ideal body weight.
   This seems to be a very popular risk factor because being over weight puts us at a higher risk.

2. Avoid or limit your intake of saturated fat from beef, pork, egg yoke, butter etc.
3. Avoid the consumption of excessive salt.
4. Minimize on your intake of alcohol.
5. Minimize on your consumption of caffeine.
6. Stay away from tobacco.
7. Eat foods rich in potassium, calcium, fish oils and magnesium.
8. Consider a daily intake of garlic, almond oil etc.

Some sources of potassium are avocados, bananas, plantain, apricot, orange, carrots, potatoes, cooked dried beans, peas and peanuts.

Sources of calcium are low fat yogurt, milk, cheese, dark green leafy vegetables, broccoli, canned fish with bones, cooked dried beans and peas. Sources of magnesium are peanuts, bananas, greens, avocado, peanut butter, cashews, low fat milk etc.

> **IN SOME CASES, HYPERTENSION MAY BE SECONDARY TO SOME DISEASES OR ABNORMALITY LEADING TO SECONDARY HYPERTENSION**

7.40 **Prevention of heart disease (cardiovascular disease)**

Cardiovascular disease is a general term for any disease of the heart and blood vessels. Heart diseases are usually caused by obstruction of the coronary arteries mainly by deposition of fat. A reduction in the flow of blood leads to chest pain, angina or even heart attack.

Causes

1. Cigarette smoking.
2. Hypertension.
3. Increase blood cholesterol levels.
4. Diabetes.
5. Obesity.
6. Excessive alcohol consumption.
7. A sedentary life style, such as waking up in the morning, taking your bath, watch television, sleep again, wake up and eat, this life style is very dangerous.
8. Lack of exercise.
9. Excessive and prolonged stress.
10. A family history of cardiovascular disease.

Signs and symptoms

1. Pain in front of the chest either on the left, centre or even on the right side.
2. Pain is increased by physical activity.
3. Pain may spread to the arms, neck, jaws or even upper part of the abdomen.
4. Difficulty in breathing and chronic in some cases.
5. Sweating is common in severe attacks.
6. Irregular heart beat in some cases.

Prevention

1. Learn how to relax and rest after work.
2. Maintain an ideal body weight.
3. Reduce the intake of foods high in fat especially saturated fats such as beef, pork, egg yokes, butter, margarine, salad dressings etc.
4. Minimize on the intake of salt or salt rich foods.
5. Reduce your intake of refined and processed sugar and foods high in sugar.
6. Increase your intake of fresh fruits and vegetables, whole grains and cereals, cooked dried beans, and peas.

7. Avoid tobacco.
8. Minimize your alcohol intake.
9. Learn how to cope with stress.
10. Ensure your bowels move regularly.
11. Do regular exercise.
12. Consider the intake of garlic daily, preferably on an empty stomach.

> **HEART DISEASES ARE USUALLY**
> **CAUSED BY OBSTRUCTION OF**
> **THE CORONARY ARTERIES**
> **MAINLY BY DEPOSITION OF FAT**

7.50   Preventing heart attack

A heart attack takes place if the flow of Oxygen-rich blood to a section of the heart muscle suddenly becomes blocked. If blood flow is not restored quickly, the section of the heart muscle will begin to die.

Causes

Heart attacks usually take place as a result of coronary heart disease (CHD), also called coronary artery disease. CHD is a condition in which a waxy substance called plaque (plak) builds up inside the coronary arteries. This plaque can be as a result of fat deposits in the arteries caused by poor diet. These arteries supply oxygen rich blood to the heart. When plaque builds up in the arteries, the condition is called atherosclerosis. This build up usually take place over many years. Eventually some part of the plaque can rupture inside an artery, this causes a blood clot to form on the plaque surface and if this blood clot becomes large enough, it can completely block blood flow through a coronary artery. And if the blockage is not treated fast, the portion of the heart muscle fed by the artery will begin to die. Healthy heart tissue is replaced with scar tissue. This can cause severe or long lasting problems.

Another rare cause of heart attack is a severe spasm (tightening) of the coronary artery. This spasm can cut off blood flow through the artery. This spasm can happen in coronary arteries not affected by plaque.

Heart attack can lead to heart failure and other problems and heart failure is a condition in which the heart cannot pump sufficient blood to meat the body's need. Arrhythmias are irregular heart beats. Ventricular fibrillation is a life threatening arrhythmia that is dangerous and can lead to death if left untreated.

Signs and Symptoms

1. Chest pain and discomfort.
2. Upper body discomfort in one or both arms, the back, neck, jaw or upper part of the stomach.
3. Shortness of breath which can happen with or before chest discomfort.
4. Nausea (feeling sick to your stomach), vomiting, light headedness or sudden dizziness or breaking out in a cold sweat.
5. Fatigue and lack of energy.
6. Sleeping problem.

Prevention

1. Follow a healthy diet; this includes a variety of fruits, vegetables, and whole grains. It also includes lean meats, poultry, fish, beans, fat free or low milk product. Your diet must be low in saturated fats, Tran's fats, cholesterol, salt and added sugar.

2. Undertake regular exercise at least 3 hours a week, this will improve your fitness level and health.

3. Stop smoking because this raises the risk of coronary heart disease.

4. Treat the condition that make heart attack more likely, such as high blood cholesterol, high blood pressure, diabetes.

5. Keep moving

   Even regular exercise is not sufficient. A study from Australia researchers found that spending more than four hours a day in front of a computer or television is associated with a doubling of serious heart problem. Prolonged sitting was found to be associated with higher levels of inflammatory marker in the blood, higher body weight and lower levels of good cholesterol (HDL). This indicates that sedentary behavior is bad for our health.

   A good remedy for heart health is getting up from your work desk every 30 minutes or even working on your computer occasionally when standing. Try taking a walk to your work colleague instead of sending an e-mail all the time. Take the stairs instead of the escalators.

6. Try not to worry, but rather devise ways to be happy. Why not try those favorite music's, films or even some of those old pictures that bring back good memories.

7. Get a good night sleep.

   Severe sleep deprivation can lead to high blood pressure, stress, risk of diabetes or fatigue.

8. Folic acid, vitamin B and hormocysteine.

   Homocysteine is chemically transformed into methionine and cysteine with the help of vitamin "B", folic acid, B12 and B6 (Pyridoxine). And a shortfall of vitamin B in the body can affect the metabolic breakdown of homocysteine and hence increase its blood levels. And high levels of homocysteine in the blood can damage the inner surface of blood vessels, which can promote blood clothing, and accelerate atherosclerosis.

The current state of knowledge regarding folic acid, homocysteine and heart attacks is as follows.

a. The level of blood folate is an important determinant of the blood homocysteine level. Low blood folate levels are associated with high blood levels of homocysteine.
b. Low blood folate is popular among individuals who do not take multivitamins.
c. The intake of folic acid supplements or folic acid fortified cereals can increase blood folate levels and decrease blood homocysteine levels.
d. In a large population study involving women, it was observed that people, who had the highest consumption of folic acid usually in the form of multivitamins, had fewer heart attacks when compared to those who consumed the least amount of folic acid.

Even though current evidence suggests that taking folic acid and vitamin B supplements to lower homocysteine levels should help prevent plaque build up and heart attacks, conclusive proof is still lacking.

9. Antioxidants that block the oxidative modification of LDL (bad cholesterol); have been shown to slow the progression of atherosclerosis in animal's experiments.
10. Example of antioxidants such as vitamin "E" and beta carotene in human observational studies have been found to lower the rate of heart attacks.

A GOOD REMEDY FOR HEART HEALTH IS GETTING UP FROM YOUR WORK DESK EVERY 30 MINUTES OR EVEN WORKING ON YOUR COMPUTER OCASSINALLY WHILE STANDING

7.60   Preventing stroke

A stroke or brain attack refers to a chemical condition where blood supply to part of the brain is suddenly or critically impaired by a blood clot (cerebral thrombosis) or when a ruptured artery leaks blood into the brain (Cerebral hemorrhage). Cerebral hemorrhage is more likely to occur in people who have high blood pressure. In either case, the affected brain cells can die from decreased blood flow and lack of oxygen.

From current studies, there are two broad categories of stroke,

1. Stroke caused by blockage of blood flow in the brain.
2. Stroke caused by ruptured artery and bleeding into the brain.

1. Stroke by blockage of blood flow in the brain.
    A blockage of blood vessel in the brain or neck, known as ischemic stroke, is the most frequent cause of stroke, and is responsible for about 30% of strokes. This blockage occurs based on three conditions.
    a. The formation of a clot within a blood vessel of the brain or neck, called thrombosis.
    b. The movement of a clot from another part of the body such as the heart to the brain, called embolism.
    c. A severe narrowing of an artery in or leading to the brain, called stenosis.

2. Stroke caused by bleeding into the brain. This is very common in people with high blood pressure and issues such as ruptured artery in the brain can lead to stroke, which is usually referred to as hemorrhagic stroke.

Causes of stroke

Each area of the brain controls a different system or part of the body and the affect of strokes depend on the part or parts of the brain the damage occurred. The situation of stroke seems to be more common in people over 50 years of age.

The common causes of stroke are,

1. High blood pressure (Hypertension).
    Hypertension increases the risk of stroke. It causes a two to four fold increase in the risk of stroke before the age of 80.

2. Cigarette smoking

    Cigarette smoking tends to cause about a two fold increase in the risk of ischemic stroke and up to four fold increase in the risk of hemorrhagic stroke. It has been linked to the accumulation of fatty substances (atherosclerosis) in the carotid artery, the main neck artery which supplies blood to the brain. Blockage of this artery is the most common cause of strokes in U.S.A. Further nicotine raises blood pressure and carbon monoxide from cigarette smoking, reduces the amount of oxygen the blood carries to the brain, coupled with the fact that smoking cigarette makes the blood thicker and more likely to clot. Smoke also increases aneurysm formation.

3. Heart disease.

    Heart disorders such as coronary artery disease, valve defects, irregular heart beat (atrial fibrillation) enlargement of one of the hearts chambers, can result in blood clots which tend to be popular in older people and is responsible for one in four strokes after the age of 80. The most popular blood vessel disease is atherosclerosis and hypertension promotes the disease and causes mechanical damages to the walls of the blood vessels.

Signs and symptoms of stroke

Warning signs of stroke are signals your body sends indicating that your brain is not receiving enough oxygen. And these are the signs to look out for before rushing to your doctor.

1. Sudden numbers or weakness of face, arm or leg, especially on one side of the body.
2. Sudden confusion or trouble talking or understanding speech.
3. Difficulty seeing in one or both eyes.
4. Difficulty walking, dizziness or loss of balance or co-ordination.
5. Sudden considerable or severe headache.

Other signs which can occur

6. Double vision.
7. Drowsiness.
8. Nausea or vomiting.
9. Paralysis of the mouth, the corner of the mouth may drop with saliva dribbling from it.

10. hot and dry skin.
11. Loss of bladder and bowel control.

Occasionally the warning signs may last only a few moments and then disappear. These brief signs known as transient ischemic attacks or TIAs, are sometimes referred to as mini strokes which indicates an underlying serious situation that needs medical attention and if ignored can be fatal and can result in death later.

Other warning signs of stroke or TIA.

1. Diabetes.

   We all think diabetes only affects our body's ability to use sugar or glucose but it also causes destructive changes in the blood vessel throughout the body, including the brain. If blood glucose levels are high at the time of stroke, the damage to the brain is usually more serious. Hypertension is popular amongst diabetic patients and accounts for more risks of stroke amongst them. Therefore treating diabetes can delay the issues of complications which tend to increase the risk of stroke.

2. Cholesterol imbalance.

   Excess low density lipoprotein (LDL) can cause cholesterol to build up in blood vessels leading to atherosclerosis, which is the major cause of the narrowing of blood vessels which can lead to stroke and heart attack.

3. Lack of exercise

   Obesity and lack of exercise is associated with hypertension, diabetes, heart disease and other disorders. Waist circumference ratio equal to or above the mid value increases the risk of ischemic stroke three fold.

Risk factors of stroke

1. Age

   Stroke occurs in any age groups, studies show that the risks double for each decade between the ages of 55 and 85. However stroke can occur in childhood and adolescence.

2. Gender

   Men have a higher risk of stroke, however more women die from stroke. Men usually do not live as long as women and tend to have stroke at a younger age which accounts for that better survival rate.

3. Race

    People from certain ethnic group have higher risk of stroke, such as people from Africa, African Americans.

4. Family history of stroke

    Stroke seems to run in some families, this can be due to an inherited issue of high blood pressure (hypertension), diabetes or an influence of there eating habits and life style.

Prevention of stroke

1. Keep your blood pressure in check (Hypertension); this is a major stroke risk if left untreated. Have blood pressure check at least yearly by your doctor or acquire and use a blood pressure monitor for your constant checks.

2. Quit smoking.

    Smoking doubles the risk of stroke. It damages blood vessels walls, speeds up the clogging of arteries, raises blood pressure and makes the heart to work harder.

3. Minimize on the use alcohol.

    Try to consume a maximum of two glasses of drink a day.

4. Keep an eye on your cholesterol level.

    The bad cholesterol (LDL) tends to clog arteries and cause stroke. Minimize on the intake of saturated fats and possibly ensure that you maintain the level of good cholesterol in your body (HDL), which tends to drain away the bad cholesterol. Eat food high in omega 3 fatty acids such as fish and consider omega 3 supplements daily.

5. Treat circulative problems.

6. Control diabetes by applying some of the issues uncovered in this book.

7. Eat a well balanced diet based on some recommendations in this book.

8. Exercise regularly at least 10 minutes a day, however 30 minutes daily is most suitable.

9. Treat transient ischemic attack (TIA.)

10. Consider drinking green tea, studies have shown that green tea can help to lower cholesterol and cut the risk of stroke.

11. Consider the use of aspirin and omega 3 supplements to prevent formation of blood clots.

12. Cut down on salts.

13. Treat your diabetes.

14. Eat fruits and vegetables.

**WARNING SIGNS OF STROKE ARE
SIGNALS YOUR BODY SENDS
INDICATING THAT YOUR BRAIN IS
NOT RECEIVING ENOUGH OXYGEN**

7.70 Preventing cancer, including prostrate cancer

Cancer

Cancer is a group of diseases characterized by the uncontrolled growth and spread of abnormal cells. The abnormal cells trespass into surrounding tissues; interfere with the tissues ability to function and eventually damage or destroy the healthy cells.

Cancer tends to develop into two stages the initiation stage and the promotion stage. The initiation stage is where the normal healthy cell or its genetic code is altered by a substance called mutagen or carcinogen.

The promotion stage is where the abnormal cell is encouraged by a substance called promoter. Studies have shown that as much as 70% of all cancers are diet related and makes diet, second only to tobacco as the most influential factor in the development of cancer.

Alcohol from studies does not initiate cancer but promotes the growth of a pre-existing abnormal cell.

Preventing cancer

1. Avoid being over weight (obesity).
    People who maintain a healthy body weight are at lower risk for developing cancers such as prostrate, uterus, gallbladder, kidney, cervix, stomach, colon and breast etc.

2. Reduce on your total fat intake, especially saturated fats.
3. Eat more high fiber foods such as whole grains, cereals, fruits and vegetables.
4. Include foods rich in vitamin A and C in your diet.
5. Include cruciferous vegetable in your diet.
6. Reduce your intake of salt, smoked and nitrite cured foods.
7. Reduce your intake of alcohol or quit entirely.
8. Stop smoking i.e. tobacco.
9. Exercise regularly.

Prostrate cancer

The prostrate is a walnut size gland in men that surrounds the urine tube. A little swelling in this small gland can cause severe urinary problem and sexual malfunction. By the age of 50 most men are at high risk of developing prostrate cancer. From studies, prostrate cancer is the leading form of male cancer.

The prostate is just below the bladder, the organ that collects and empties urine and in front of the rectum, the lower part of the intestine. The prostrate gland produces fluid that make up part of the semen. In fact prostrate cancer is a disease in which malignant (cancer) cells form in the tissues of the prostrate. As men age, the prostrate may get bigger. A bigger prostrate may block the flow of urine from the bladder and cause problem with sexual function. This condition is called benign prostatic hyperplasia (BPH). This is not cancerous, but surgery is necessary to correct it in most circumstances. The symptoms of BPH are equivalent to most problems in prostrate cancer.

The usual medical treatment for prostrate cancer is surgery, radiation, microwave, toxic dust, including chemotherapy. Men should have their prostrate specific antigen (PSA) and prostrate acid phosphatase (PAP) levels checked every year, especially if you are 50 years and above.

Signs and symptom

1. Difficulty in urinating.
2. Inability to empty the bladder completely.
3. Pain when urinating.
4. Pain during sex.
5. Need to get up in the night to urinate sometimes in a number of occasions.

Prevention of prostrate cancer

1. Healthy diet

A healthy diet low in fat and full of fruits and vegetables is recommended. Especially diet low in saturated fats. Foods that tend to contain fats of this nature include meats, dairy products such as milk and cheese. You should concentrate on eating more fats from plants than animals. For instance cook with olive oil, rather than butter, sprinkle nuts in your salads rather than cheese.

Increase the amounts of fruits and vegetables you eat.

2. **Eat fish**

   Fatty fish such as salmon, sardines, tuna, trout which contain omega-3 fatty acids, has been lnked to reduce prostrate cancer.

3. **Reduce the amount of dairy products you eat daily**

   This includes milk, cheese yogurt. Go for a low fat equivalent.

4. **Drink green tea**

   Some studies show that it reduces prostrate cancer risk.

5. **Add soy to your diet**

   Diets that include tofu, a product made from soy bean have been linked to a reduced risk of prostrate cancer. Also try soy milk instead of animal milk. The benefit of soy comes from a specific nutrient called isoflavones. Other sources of isoflavones are kidney beans, chick peas, lentils peanuts and many others.

6. **Reduce your alcohol intake**
7. **Maintain a healthy weight**

   Men with a body mass index (BMI) of 30 and above are considered obese and tend to have high prostrate cancer risk.

8. Exercise regularly
9. Talk to your doctor about your risks
10. Stop smoking

BY THE AGE OF 50 MOST MEN ARE AT HIGHER RISK OF DEVELOPING PROSTRATE CANCER

7.80   <u>Stomach ulcer (peptic ulcer) and prevention</u>

Any ulcer in the digestive system is known as peptic ulcer. This includes both gastric (occurring in stomach) and duodenal ulcers. These are very common in middle aged men and women, who tend to be acidity patients. The ulcers are formed when a small area of the stomach or duodenal lining loses its natural resistance to the acids and other juices involved in the digestive process. When this occurs, the acids and digestive juices erode the weak point of the lining and create a sore patch which leads to the formation of ulcer. An ulcer is not contagious or cancerous.

The size of a stomach ulcer can range between 12.5% of an inch to 75% of an inch.

<u>Causes</u>

1. Destruction of the gastric or intestinal mucosal lining of the stomach, by hydrochloric acid, present in the digestive juices of the stomach.
2. Infection with the bacterium helicobacter pylori, which can be transmitted from person to person through contaminated food and water. Antibiotics are the most effective treatment.
3. Injury of the gastric mucosal lining and weakening of the mucous defenses.
4. Excessive secretion of hydrochloric acid.
5. Genetic predisposition.
6. Stress.
7. Chronic use of anti-inflammatory drugs such as aspirin.
8. Cigarette smoking.
9. Heavy drinking.
10. Not having regular meals.
11. Excessive hot and spicy foods.
12. Excessive tea and coffee.
13. Pan chewing etc.

<u>Signs and symptoms</u>

1. Burning feeling in the stomach that lasts between 30 minutes and 3 hours.
2. Indigestion or hunger.
3. Pain in the upper abdomen, but occasionally below the breast bone. In some people pain occurs immediately after eating and in some cases hours after eating. Pains usually awakens the person at night, weeks of pain may be followed by weeks of not having pain.

What stomach ulcer affect

1. Nerves surrounding the stomach.

   The nerves become agitated and cause severe pain. Stomach ulcer can cause hemorrhage from the erosion of a major blood vessel, a tear in the wall of the stomach or intestine, with resultant peritonitis or obstruction of the gastrointestinal track, because of spasm or swelling in the areas of ulcer.

Prevention and treatment

1. Eat breakfast and other meals regularly.
2. Avoid hot spicy foods.
3. Stop smoking.
4. Manage your stress.
5. Drink alcohol in moderation and not in an empty stomach.
6. Minimize in your use of anti-inflammatory drugs such as aspirin etc.
7. Banana fruits contain some ulcer healing properties.
8. Honeys tend to ease the pain.

Risks of developing stomach ulcer

1. Family history of the disease.
2. Smoking.
3. Excessive alcohol intake.
4. Excessive use of anti-inflammatory drugs such as aspirin.
5. Zollinger-Ellison syndrome.
6. Improper diet, irregular or skipped meals.
7. Drinking alcohol on empty stomach.
8. Type O, blood (for duodenal ulcers).
9. Stress
10. Chromic disorder such as liver disease, emphysema, rheumatoid arthritis, may increase vulnerability.

> **THE SIZE OF STOMACH**
> **ULCER CAN RANGE**
> **BETWEEN 12.5% OF AN INCH**
> **TO 75% OF AN INCH**

7.90   Preventing Heart burn

Heart burn is a burning or painful sensation in the stomach or upper end of the stomach located near the heart. Heart burn can be due to increased stomach acid or crowded conditions inside the abdomen.

Heart burn overview

The esophagus is a tube that connects the mouth to the stomach. It is made of muscles that work to push food towards the stomach in rhythmic waves. Once in the stomach, food is prevented from refluxing, that is moving back into the esophagus by a special area of circular muscle located at the junction of the esophagus and stomach, called the lower esophageal sphincter (LES). A pressure difference across the diaphragm, the flat muscle that separates the chest from the abdomen, also tends to keep stomach contents in the stomach.

The stomach combines food, acids and enzymes together to start the process of digestion. There are special protective cells that line the stomach to prevent the acid from causing inflammation. The esophagus lacks this same protection and if stomach products reflux back into the esophagus; this can cause inflammation to the lining.

Heartburn is caused by acid refluxing back into the esophagus, and tends to be more pronounced for those that increase the production of acid in the stomach.

Causes of heart burn

1. Some popular food we eat and drink, including over the counter prescription drugs can stimulate increase stomach acid secretion, which results in heart burn.

Some examples are,

   a. Caffeine.
   b. Aspirin.
   c. Alcohol.
   d. Other anti-inflammatory drugs such as Ibuprofen, nuprin.
   e. Carbonated beverages.
   f. Acid juices such as grapefruits, orange, pineapples and tomatoes.
   g. Chocolate.

2. Smoking
3. Consumption of foods high in fat contents.
4. A hiatal hernia, in which a portion of the stomach lies in the chest instead of the abdomen, hiatal hernia cause no symptoms, it is only when the LES falls, that heart burn begins.
5. Pregnancy can cause increased pressure in the abdomen and hence cause heart burn.
6. Similarly obesity can increase heart burn, due to increased pressure in the abdomen.
7. Primary disease of the esophagus can also cause heart burn these include, scleroderma, sarcoidesis etc.

Prevention of heart burn

1. Eat reduced and more frequent meals.
   This is because over eating tends to put extra pressure on the lower esophagus sphincter (LES) and increase the chances of a heart burn.

2. Minimize or stay away from foods and beverages that tend to trigger reflux of stomach contents, some of these are cola drink, carbonated beverages, citrus fruits and juices, tomatoes, chocolates, spicy and fatty foods, alcohol, coffee and tea.
3. Avoid eating within two to three hours before bed time. Lying down with a full stomach tend to cause the contents of the stomach to press harder against the LES and increase the chances of refluxed food leading to heart burn.
4. Reduce your weight if you are obese. Obesity increases abnormal pressures leading to heart burn.
5. Elevate your head a few inches while you sleep, lying down flat presses the stomach contents against the LES, and leading to heart burn.
6. Avoid wearing belts or clothes that are tight around the waist. This habit tends to squeeze the stomach, hence forcing food up against the LES, leading to heart burn.
7. Stop smoking
   Chemicals in cigarettes weaken the LES, as they pass from the lungs into the blood.

8. Avoid alcohol.

   This tends to increase the production of stomach acid. However if you cannot cope, dilute your alcohol intake with water or sugar free soft drinks. Alcohol also relaxes the lower esophageal sphincter, hence allowing the reflux of stomach contents into the esophagus.

9. Keep a heart burn record.

   Recording what triggers your heart burn will help you keep a check on your heart burn and avoid this situation.

10. Take your medication at the some time every day.

11. Avoid commercial antacids made with anything other than calcium. Calcium is natures own antacid, it neutralizes excess stomach acid and help the digestive system function better. Milk product, yogurt are good sources of calcium.

THE STOMACH COMBINES FOOD, ACIDS AND ENZYMES TOGETHER TO START THE PROCESS OF DIGESTION

7.100 <u>Preventing diabetes</u>

<u>Diabetes mellitus</u>

Diabetes is characterized by a reduced ability to use and metabolize dietary carbohydrates, elevated blood sugar levels, and abnormal amount of sugar in the urine.

There are two types,

1. Type 1 diabetes, called insulin dependent diabetes (IDDM); this is also called juvenile onset diabetes.
2. Type 2 diabetes called no insulin dependent diabetes (NIDDM); it is also called adult onset diabetes, when the cells of the pancreas are weak.

1. <u>Type 1 Diabetes (Insulin dependant diabetes (IDDM)</u>

This type of diabetes occurs when the body produces virtually no insulin. This usually develops in the early teens though it can occur later in life. It usually develops very fast, often over a few days.

<u>Signs and symptoms</u>

Feeling of weakness, severe thirsty feeling, passage of large amount of urine, rapid loss of weight because the body is unable to use or store its glucose, the body draws on its stores of fat or energy, confusion or sleepiness. Without prompt treatment, the condition can become severe and the person can lose consciousness and pass into a diabetic coma, the breath may smell of alcohol.

2. <u>Types 2 Diabetes non insulin dependent diabetes (NIDDM)</u>

It is a milder form, resulting when the body produces some insulin but not enough for its needs. Most people in this group are usually over 40 years and over weight.

<u>Signs and symptoms</u>

Initial symptom of thirst, excessive urine usually occurs over some months by gradual onset, tiredness, feeling of pins and needles, blurred vision.

<u>General causes of diabetes</u>

1. Over weight.
2. Lack of exercise.

3. Excess fat.
4. Poor diet.
5. Lack of hormone insulin.

   When we consume things such as bread, cakes, biscuits and foods containing sugar and starch, the digestive process in the bowel break down the sugar and starch into glucose, which is absorbed into the blood stream. Insulin is produced in the pancreas and assists the body to process the glucose in the blood so that it can be used for fuel, muscle activity and other body functions. After processing, any excess can be stored in the liver as glycogen, to be converted later into energy or fat. In diabetic patients, the pancreas does not produce enough insulin to allow the glucose in the blood to be used. In some situation no insulin is produced.

6. Heredity, history of diabetes that runs in the family.
7. Age, which can cause the pancreas to become inefficient.

Prevention of diabetes

1. Maintain an ideal body weight; about 3 out of 4 diabetic patients are over weight.
2. Eat diet high in whole grains and cereals, fruits, vegetables, cooked dry beans, peas, potatoes and unrefined starch.
3. Vitamins and minerals from fruits, vegetables, multivitamin supplements that contains all the vitamins and most of the minerals especially chromium and magnesium, helps in the prevention and treatment of diabetes.
4. Regular exercise improves how the body uses insulin and helps in the regulation of blood sugar levels. Aerobic exercise, jogging, stationary or out door, cycling performed 3 to 4 times a week for 20 minutes or more tends to assist in overall lowering effect of blood sugar.

IN DIABETIC PATIENTS, THE PANCREAS DOES NOT PRODUCE ENOUGH INSULIN TO ALLOW THE GLUCOSE IN THE BLOOD TO BE USED

CHAPTER 8

8.00   Some medical foods and their healing qualities

Some foods have some good healing qualities; some are also characterized with super healing qualities and contributes to a youthful look.

8.10   Foods with super-healing qualities

a. Cherries.
b. Guavas.
c. Beans.
d. Kiwifruit.
e. Watercress.
f. Spinach.
g. Onions.
h. Carrots.
i. Cabbage.
j. Broccoli.

a. Cherries

Cherries are full of substances that help fight inflammation and cancer. Quercetin and ellagic acid which are two compounds found in cherries have been found to inhibit the growth of tumors and even destroy cancer cell without damaging healthy cells. They also have antiviral and antibacterial properties. Anthocyanin, a compound found in cherries tends to lower the Uric acid levels in the blood which subsequently reduce the common cause of gout. Studies show that it reduces the risk of colon cancer. The substances also work as a natural form of Ibuprofen and reduce inflammation and pain. If taken regularly, cherries may assist in the lowering of the risk of heart attack and stroke.

b. Guavas

Guavas contain a cancer fighting antioxidant lycopene. They seem to have more of this than any other fruit or vegetable. Tomatoes also contain this antioxidant, but our body tends to struggle with processing it unless they are cooked, the processing helps break breakdown tough cell walls. However, guavas cell structure allows the antioxidant to be absorbed easily in a raw or cooked form and offers the nutrition without the added sodium of processed tomato products.

Lycopene protects our healthy cells from free radicals that can cause different kinds of damage, including blocking arteries, joint degeneration, nervous system malfunction, and cancer. Lycopene intake is associated with low rates of prostrate cancer; it is also associated with considerable improvement in the reduction of prostrate tumors. They are also found to inhibit the growth of breast cancer cells and studies show that they help protect against coronary heart disease.

Guavas are also full of vitamin C and other antioxidants. Guavas also offer more than 60% more potassium than bananas, which can help protect against heart disease and stroke. The nutrient found in guava have been shown to lower LDL and increase HDL Cholesterol, reduce triglycerides and lower blood pressure. One or two guavas a day is very good. Most guava juices are processed and sweetened and will not provide the same superior nutrition from the fruit itself.

c. Beans

Beans tend to lower cholesterol, regulate blood sugar and insulin production, promotes digestive health and guards against cancer. Beans tend to be associated with the phrase three in one, because of its fiber, protein and antioxidants content. Which can cover us for whole grain, meat and fruit in the real sense of it.

An assortment of phytochemicals found in beans has been linked to the protection of cells from cancerous activity by stopping cancer cells from reproducing and slowing tumor growth. Studies from Harvard school of public health found that women who consumed beans at least two times a weak were 24% less likely to develop breast cancer and several studies have linked beans to a reduced risk of heart disease, type 2 diabetes, high blood pressure, breast and colon cancer.

Beans have a high amount of antioxidants which help to prevent and tackle oxidative damage. Studies have placed three varieties of beans to be very high in antioxidants, red beans, red kidney beans, and pinto beans. Other beans are also equally good. Beans are also good sources of iron. They further contain amino acid tryptophan, foods with high volume of tryptophan tend to help regulate appetite, aid in sleep and improve our mood. They are also reach in folate, which is good for the heart.

And depending on your choice of beans, you can get a good amount of potassium, magnesium, vitamin B1 and B2, vitamin K. Soya beans is a good source of omega-3 fatty acids.

In Chinese traditional medicine some types of beans have been linked to the treatment of food poisoning, edema, high blood pressure, diarrhea, kidney stones, laryngitis, rheumatism etc.

Adzuki and mung beans are easily digested. Pinto, kidney, navy, garbanzo, lemma and black beans are more difficult to digest.

d. Kiwi fruit

This fruit has a high amount of vitamin C, in fact twice the amount found in oranges. It has more fiber than apples and is higher in potassium than banana. The blend of phytonutrients, vitamins and mineral in kiwi fruits helps in the protection against heart disease, stroke, cancer and respiratory disorders. Kiwi fruits have a natural blood thinning properties, which works with no side effects like aspirin. It is good for vascular health and reduces the formation of spontaneous blood clots, lowers LDL Cholesterol and blood pressure. Studies have also shown that it reduces oxidative stress and damage to DNA and encourages damaged cells to repair themselves. We must aim to eat one to two kiwi fruit a day. The riper the kiwi fruit the more the antioxidant power.

e. Water cress

It is close enough as a calorie free food. It provides around four times the calcium of 2% milk, offers as much vitamin C as orange and more iron than spinach. It also has lots of vitamin A and also vitamin K along with multiple antioxidants, carotenoids and protective phytochemicals.

Its nutrients protect against cancer and macular degeneration, boost immune system and supports bone health. Its iron helps the red blood cells to carry oxygen to the body tissues for energy. The phytochemicals in water cress tackles cancer in 3 ways; it kills the cells, blocking carcinogens and protects healthy cells from carcinogens. They also help in the prevention of lung and esophageal cancer and other cancers. Water cress is best when eaten raw although it can be cooked. In Chinese medicine it is used to reduce tumors, improve night vision, stimulate bile production, hence improving digestion and setting intestinal gas, remedy for jaundice, urinary problem, sore throat, mumps and bad breath etc.

f. Spinach

Spinach protects against eye disease and loss of vision and it is good for brain function. It protects against colon, prostrate and breast cancer, including heart disease, stroke, dementia, lowers blood pressure, anti-inflammatory and good for the bone. Spinach has high nutrients of vitamin K, calcium, vitamin A, vitamin C, folate, magnesium and iron.

Carotenoid found in spinach kills prostrate cancer cells and prevents them from multiplying; folate boosts vascular health by lowering homocysteine, an amino acid when high increases the risk of dementia, heart disease and stroke. Folate also reduces the risk of developing colorectal, ovarian and breast cancers and assists in the stopping of uncontrolled cell growth which is one of the main characteristics of all cancers. The vitamin C and beta-carotene in spinach protects against colon cancer, fights inflammation, which makes them a vital component of brain health, especially in older generation.

Spinach has a lot of vitamin K for strong bones, they are also reach in lutein which guards against age related degeneration and can help prevent heart attacks by keeping artery walls clear of cholesterol build up. Spinach is best eaten lightly steamed or raw. Conventionally grown spinach is prone to pesticide residue, it is better to go for the organic type.

g. Onions

Onions has a good cancer fighting enzymes. Its consumption helps to lower the risk of prostrate and esophageal cancers and guards against coronary heart disease. Studies have also shown that they may help in the prevention of stomach cancer.

Onions contains sulfides that help to lower blood pressure and cholesterol. It also has peptide that can help to prevent bone loss. Onions has super antioxidant power, they contain quercetin, a natural antihistamine that reduces airway inflammation and assists in the relief of symptoms of allergies and hay fever. It also has a high amount of vitamin C which together with quercetin battles cold and flu symptoms, its anti-inflammatory properties helps to fight the pain and swelling associated with osteo and rheumatoid arthritis. They are very rich in sulfur and have antibiotic and antiviral properties, making onions very good for people who consume a diet high in protein, fat or sugar because they help to cleanse the arteries and stop the growth of viruses, yeasts and other disease causing agents, which can build up an imbalance diet.

It is good to eat onion once a day or half, preferably raw, although you can cook it lightly. Onion tends to reduce carcinogens produced by the meat we eat.

h. Carrots

They are good sources of potent antioxidants known as carotenoids. Diets high in carotenoids have been linked to a decreased risk of post menopausal breast cancer including cancer of the bladder, cervix, prostrate, colon, larynx and esophagus. Also diets low in carotenoids has been linked with various cancers and heart disease. Studies have shown that just one carrot a day can reduce your risk of lung cancer by 50%. It may also reduce your risk of ovarian and kidney cancers. Not only does carrot fight cancer, the nutrients in carrots prevent cardiovascular disease, stimulate the immune system, and supports colon, ear and eye health.

Carrots contain calcium, potassium, magnesium, phosphorus, fiber, vitamin C and a very high amount of vitamin A. The alpha-carotene in carrots is linked to the prevention of tumor growth. They also contain carotenoids lutein and zeaxanthin, which work together to promote eye health and prevent macular degeneration and cataracts.

In Chinese medicine carrot are used to treat rheumatism, kidney stone, tumors, indigestion, diarrhea, night blindness, ear infections, deafness, skin lesions, urinary track infections, coughs and constipation.

It is good to eat carrot raw or lightly cooked. Cooking helps breakdown the tough fiber making some of the nutrients easier to absorb.

Remove carrots tips before storing them in the fridge, because the tips draw moisture from the root, hence causing the carrot to wilt.

i. Cabbage

Cabbage contains a high amount of vitamin K, and C, it also has good amount of fiber, manganese, vitamin B6 and folate.

It has high levels of antioxidant sulforaphanes that fight free radicals before they damage DNA; they also stimulate enzymes that detoxify Carcinogens in the body. Studies show that this ability may account to their ability to reduce the risk of cancer more effectively than any other plant food group. A lot of studies points to the association between diets high in cruciferous vegetables such as cabbage and the link to a reduced lung, colon, breast, ovarian and bladder cancers.

Cabbage promotes strong bones, reduces inflammation and promotes good gastrointestinal health. It is commonly used in a juiced form, as a natural remedy for healing peptic ulcers.

It provides significant cardiovascular benefit by preventing plaque formation in the blood vessels.

In Chinese medicine, cabbage is used to treat constipation, common cold, whooping cough, depression, stomach ulcers. When eaten and used as a poultice, cabbage is helpful for healing bedsores, varicose veins and arthritis.

The higher the cabbage in your diet, the better. Red cabbage are far superior to the white ones with about seven times more vitamin C and more than four times the polypheriols which protect cells from oxidative stress and cancer. However both are nutritional stars.

j. Broccoli

A single cut of steamed broccoli provides more than 200% of the RDA for vitamin C, nearly as much as vitamin K, and about half of the daily allowance for vitamin A, coupled with a lot of folate, fiber, sulfur, iron and vitamins B. Broccoli contains about twice the amount of protein as steak and a lot more protective phytonutrients. Broccolis phytochemicals fight cancer by neutralizing carcinogens and accelerating their elimination from the body. Besides preventing tumors caused by chemical carcinogens, they also help prevent esophageal cancers and other cancers.

Phytonutrients called indoles found in broccoli, help protect against prostrate, gastric, skin, breast and cervical cancers. Many studies have also linked broccoli to a 20% reduction in heart disease.

In Chinese medicine, broccoli is used to treat eye inflammation.

You will be doing your body a favor if you can eat broccoli every day. If you cannot manage it, try eating it at least twice a week. Cooking broccoli reduces some of the anticancer components, you are advised to lightly steam broccoli to preserve most of the nutrients.

Other foods and their healing qualities

1. Chili pepper

The source of heat in chilies is an antioxidant which can protect the body against carcinogen. It is also a natural decongestant and expectorant. Its blood thinning ability helps to prevent strokes, it also lowers cholesterol.

2. Red pepper

It can be of good use for digestive and pain reliever. In digestive aid, it assists in the stimulation of stomach secretions and saliva. It contains capsaicin, the pain reliever (analgesic). It has often been used for the treatment of shingles, diabetic foot pain and cluster headache.

3. Tomatoes or strawberries

In a study of plants that give longevity, researches found that the two that best provide the highest result for longer life were tomatoes and strawberries. Tomatoes are rich in lycopenes an antioxidant that stimulates immune system function and slows degenerative diseases. Tomatoes are rich in vitamin C and A, and have low fat and sodium. They also contain fiber and potassium. Some studies also show that tomatoes tend to soak up molecules in the brain that can damage cells.

Graham A. Coldtiz M.D and his associates at Harvard medical school discovered that the chances of dying of cancer were lowest among those who ate tomatoes and strawberries every week. Strawberries contain ellagic acid, which have been shown to contain anti-cancer properties.

4. Pineapple

Pineapple is rich in manganese, which is the essential part of certain enzymes needed to metabolize protein and carbohydrates. It has no sodium and fat content. Enzymes, the catalyst that speed up the rate of reaction in the body are found in high amount in pineapple, which help combat things like, auto immune disease, allergies and cancer.

5. Pawpaw (papaya)

Ripe papaya is rich in vitamin A and C. In traditional medicine the milky fluid known as latex is used to treat psoriasis, ring worm, and other skin disorders. The unripe papaya is also used to trigger menstruation. The ripe one also helps in digestion and prevents ulcer.

6. Mangoes

Mango is rich in caroteniods. They also contain bioflavonoid, they aid the immune system. Mangoes make the grade of more than a days worth of vitamin A, carotene, with 30% recommended dietary allowance. This vitamin A also comes with the full allowance of vitamin C too.

7. Garlic

Garlic is a power house of antioxidant of various kinds. It lowers cholesterol and blood pressure. It is an antiviral and anti bacterial and may have chemicals capable of destroying cancer cells. Garlic is used by Indians to treat infections, wound, cancer, digestive problems, common cold, epilepsy, cough and whooping cough. Most modern physician recommend garlic for colds, cough, flu, fever, bronchitis, heart diseases, stroke, liver and gall bladder disorder, lead poisoning and diabetes. Garlic increases immune functions.

8. Mushrooms

A particular type of hard woody mushrooms that grow on tree trunks, contain beta-glucan which acts like a vaccine to kick start the immune system at a higher speed. They also have anticancer and anti-viral properties. It must be noted that it is not good to pick and eat wild mushrooms.

9. Citrus fruits

Fresh citrus fruits are a great source of vitamin C. Several studies have linked this fruit in fighting cancer of the lungs, cervix, esophagus and stomach cancer. They are very rich in bioflavonoids.

10. Bananas

Bananas contain a significant amount of soluble fiber. It is high in potassium, which helps to control blood pressure. Lack of potassium in the body tends to cause high and low blood pressure. Bananas are rich in vitamin C; they also have high magnesium content, which helps to protect the circulatory system. The pectin content of bananas, which is a soluble fiber, prevents radical swings in blood sugar.

11. Soy Beans

Soy bean, soya milk and soy protein reduces low density lipo protein (LDL), the bad cholesterol and hence reduces heart disease risk. Soy is further rich in phyto-estrogen, a category of bioflavonoid that inhibits estrogen promoting cancer. It also protects against radiation in chemotherapy. Research show that soy eaters have reduced risk of prostrate, colon, lung, rectal and stomach cancers.

They contain multiple cancer fighting compounds. Genistein found only in soybean has the ability to block the development of cancer in several different stages. They play a preventive role for diabetes, gall bladder, kidney stones, premenstrual symptoms, menopausal symptoms, high blood pressure, cancer and heart diseases.

12. Fish

Fish tend to be low in fat and high in omega 3 fatty acids which reduce the risk of heart disease and cancer. Fish contains very little saturated fat and is a cholesterol lowering diet.

Fish such as mackerel, sable fish, white fish, salmon, tuna etc, contain a high level of omega 3 fatty acids which helps to prevent blood pressure because of the potassium content. They also make the blood less prone to clotting, which can lead to heart attack or stroke. Fish prevents heart disease.

British scientist J.M. Kremer also found in his studies, that omega 3 fatty acids found in fish helps to reduce inflammation by helping the body make substance known as prostaglandin, which tend to reduce inflammation. The omega 3 fatty acids are good for treating rheumatoid arthritis. They also protect against age related mental decline, loss of cognitive function usually associated with aging.

13. Grape fruit

Grape fruit is high in vitamin C, and has pectin, a kind of fiber found in grape fruit. Dr. James Cerda M.D of the University of Florida in his studies on pectin discovered that grape fruit is good for keeping the heart healthy. It has low fat and sodium but is rich in potassium which helps to lower the blood pressure.

14. Oats and Bran

Oats are high in fiber and have no fat and sodium in detectable level. James W. Anderson, a professor at the University of Kentucky college of medicine, found that the high fiber oats diet he developed for his diabetic patients were bringing down their insulin level and blood cholesterol level.

Oats reduces the insulin level in the blood which subsequently prevents diabetes. Oats also reduces the cholesterol level in the blood which subsequently prevents high blood pressure.

15. Oranges

Oranges are high in vitamin C and low in fat and sodium. And it is a very powerful antioxidant.

16. Apples

An apple a day tends to keep you away from the Doctors. Apple has pectin the type of fiber also found in banana. Pectin is a soluble fiber that has the ability of lowering high blood pressure, reduces the risk of heart disease, heart failure, diabetes, constipation, cancer, diarrhea and rheumatism.

Pectin also helps to eliminate toxic materials from the body, such as lead and mercury.

Eat all fresh apples, but stay away from the seeds inside.

17. Avocado Pears

Pears are low in fat and sodium and rich in insoluble fibers, which aid the digestive health. Avocado pears are good for peptic ulcer, hypertension, insomnia and gastro intestinal problems.

Avocado Seed

The seed of avocado is rich in nutrition and can be medicinal. You can grind it in a high powered blender of food processor for use in smoothies and other foods.

In Chinese and African medicine the grinded avocado seed, is usually dried in the sun and the powder preserved and use for treating high blood pressure. Two tea spoonfuls are usually mixed with pap or taken directly once a day until the symptoms of high blood pressure disappears.

Avocado Seed has the following Healing Properties

1. Anti-tumor properties.

   While human studies are yet to confirm this, however test in rats and mice indicate that compounds in the seed has anti-tumor properties.

   According to the Encyclopedia of common natural ingredients used in food, drugs and cosmetics, an avocado seed has a condensed flavonoid that is responsible for anti-tumor.

2. Antioxidant Properties

A 2003 study at the National University of Singapore concluded that avocado seed, among other fruits including mango, tamarind and jackfruit have an even greater level of antioxidant activity than the more commonly eaten parts of the fruits. The seed may contain more than 70% of the antioxidants found in the fruit.

3. Digestive Properties

American Indians used avocado seed to treat both dysentery and diarrhea.

4. Soluble Fiber

The avocado seed is among the highest naturally occurring sources of soluble fiber, which helps to lower cholesterol levels.

5. Potassium

A 1951 article by the California Avocado Society indicates that avocado seeds are very high in potassium. However the level of potassium declines as the fruit mature. These properties are very good for lowering high blood pressure. Sufficient levels of phosphorus are also present in the seed.

18. Bran Wheat

Bran wheat is loaded with fiber, iron and potassium. It is low in sodium and it is a good source of vitamin B. It also has a significant amount of protein. Bran wheat is good for preventing diversticular diseases, digestive disorders, constipation and irritable bowel syndrome.

19. Barley

Barley is a low fat food. It is rich in fiber and protein, with low sodium. It is very good for those who want to lose weight.

20. Cereals

Cereals come in many forms, oat bran dry, corn bran, puffed wheat, oat flak. Cereals are good for the treatment of diabetic patients.

21. Corn

Corn is loaded with minerals such as iron, zinc, and potassium. They are low in sodium and have a significant amount of protein. People who live in beans and corn rarely suffer high blood cholesterol and hardening of arteries.

22. Lemon

Lemon contains vitamin B1, B2 and C. it also contains flavonoids and organic acids. They are good for indigestion, scurvy, sore throat and kidney stone. It can prevent and dissolve kidney stones and cancer. They also improve blood circulation and are good for hypertension; heart problems and stroke. Lemon juice also cleanses and rejuvenates the cells, organs and tissues in the body. Ulcer patients should avoid lemon juice.

23. Lettuce

Lettuce has a high level of carotene, some vitamin C, and a little trace of fat and sodium. They are good in fighting cancer.

24. Coconut

The water in coconut is an excellent cleanser. It is also a good antibody. It strengthens the immune system to resist illnesses. Coconut is also used to neutralize the effects of hard drugs or overdose. In traditional medicine, the immature white pulp of coconut is used by people suffering from memory loss or forgetfulness.

25. Melon

Melon comes in many types such as water melon, cantaloupe, casaba and honeydew. Melon is rich in vitamin C and is a good source of potassium, which helps in reducing blood pressure. Also studies by Regina G. Zigler and her associates at National Cancer Institute USA, found a link between melon intake and other similar vitamins, and protection from cancer of the esophagus.

26. Low Fat Milk

Drinking low fat milk is better than the one with high fat, preferably skim milk. A low fat milk is better for blood pressure. It is also better for bone health. Aging people are better off drinking milk to boost their bone health because of its high calcium content.

27. Millet

Millet increases your intake of the protective trio of carbohydrates, fiber, vegetable and protein. Millet is good for the heart health and protects it from heart diseases.

28. Potatoes

Potatoes are very rich in fiber and potassium. You must not boil potatoes because 10 to 50% of its potassium content may be lost. It is better to steam potatoes to maintain the nutritional contents. Potatoes help to lower cholesterol due to its fiber contents. It helps to lower blood pressure due to its potassium contents.

29. Pumpkin

Pumpkin is a high fiber food with a lot of vitamin A and a high level of beta-carotene, which are good nutrients for cancer prevention. They are also rich in minerals such as calcium, magnesium, copper and zinc.

30. Plantain

Plantain rates higher than bananas for vitamin A and potassium. They are both low in sodium and fat. They are also rich in fiber.

Plantain due to its potassium contents lowers blood pressure. It also keeps the heart healthy.

Unripe plantain is a healing food for diabetic patients.

31. Peas

Peas tend to keep the heart healthy since they have little or no fat, cholesterol and sodium. They help to control diabetes, because of their high fiber content and low fat. Peas also help in the prevention of cancer because of the fiber content together with its carotene and vitamin C plus low fat content.

32. Raspberry

Raspberry leaves and fruits are used to treat diarrhea, fever, ulcer, putrid sores of the mouth, piles, kidney stones and heavy menstrual flow in traditional medicines. In traditional medicine, it is usually referred to as the herb for pregnant women.

33. Bread

White bread made of flour is fattening food, and is not good for our health, however whole wheat bread is good in boosting our health. The benefits of whole wheat bread include;

a. The bread is good for people who want to lose weight
b. Because wheat bread is rich in complex carbohydrates and fiber, it is good in reducing blood cholesterol and it is recommended by most experts for the reduction in cancer risks.
c. It also facilitates good digestive health.

34. Green

Green are rich in vitamin A as carotene, they are also good fiber foods and low in fat. They are good in lowering cholesterol, prevention of cancer, and good in controlling diabetes. However you must not overcook green, it is best cooked half done.

35. Green Beans

Green beans are a good source of fiber, iron and potassium and tend to be low in fat and sodium. The high potassium and fiber contents are good in lowering blood pressure.

36. Ginger

In Chinese traditional medicine, ginger is used to treat kidney problems and arthritis. Chinese women still drink ginger tea for menstrual cramps, morning sickness, cold flu, heart disease and stroke.

37. Sweet potato

Sweet potatoes are very rich in vitamin A; they also have high carotene content and are very good for cancer prevention especially lung cancer.

38. Tangerines

Like oranges, tangerines are good for their vitamin C content; it also has a good amount of vitamin A. They are good for reducing fat and helps in maintaining weight. They offer most of the advantages found in oranges.

39. Brown rice

Brown rice is good because it provides all the fiber and nutrients that nature put in the grain. It also has some protein contents and is good for high blood pressure.

40. Sage

The ancient Greeks and Romans used sage as a meat preservative. They also used sage to treat snake bite, intestinal worms, chest ailments and menstrual problems. Sage is used for longevity by the Arabs and Italians and the French use it for nerve stimulation. Hundreds of years ago, people from Iceland used it for bladder infections and kidney stones. In Chinese medicine, sage is used to treat insomnia, depression, gastrointestinal disorders, menstrual problems and nipple inflammation in nursing mothers.

41. Cassava

In Africa, most farmers rely on eating cassava raw after snake bite in the bush before getting proper medical attention. The raw cassava tend to neutralize the Vernon long enough to receive treatment.

42. Bitter leaf

Bitter leaf contains vernodalin, venomygolin and saponin. In Africa traditional medicine its juice is used as a remedy to cure stomach ache, skin infection. It is also used as an aid in the prevention of diabetes and stroke.

43. Bitter Kola

Bitter Kola contains kolaviron, flavonoids, tannins and resin. In Africa it is used as an anti-poison for snake bite, food poison or any other poison when chewed in empty stomach. It is also used as a remedy for jaundice and hepatitis in Africa.

44. Kola

West African slaves introduced the kola tree into Brazil and Caribbean. In African traditional medicine, it is used to treat, water retention, digestive problems, diarrhea, pneumonia and attempt to break the tobacco habit.

CONCLUSION

I belief that a lot of facts uncovered from this work will go a long way in assisting a lot of individuals in some of the decision they make in their daily eating habits and life style. I hope that some of these ideas will serve as a waking up call which will be the first step for most people in making that vital decision in their way of life. It must be noted that, it is always very difficult to make that, first vital decision and even more difficult to pursue that goal even after making the decision. I believe it is all about self control and determination and most importantly being able to acknowledge the immense benefits that will accrue in taking that bold step particularly many years down the line.

REFERENCES

1. PDR for Herbal supplements. 2nd Ed
   Medical Economics 2008.
2. Textbook of Nutritional Medicine
   Melvyn werbach and Jeffery Moss Third Line Press Tarzana California 1999.
3. PDR for Nutritional Supplements
   Medical Economics 2001.
4. Nutrition for Injury Rehabilitation and Sports Medicine.
   Luke Bucci. CRC Press Boca Raton Florida 1995.
5. Clinical Nutrition, a Functional Approach.
   Institute for Functional Medical Inc. Gig Harbor Washington 1999
6. Advanced Human Nutrition.
   Robert Wildman and Denis Medeiros CRC Press
   Boca Raton, Florida 2000.
7. Amino Acids and Proteins for the Athlete.
   Mario Di Pasquale CRC Press Boca Raton Florida 1997.
8. Nutritional Influence on Illness.
   Second Edition Melvyn Werbach, Michael Murray. Third Line Press Tarzana, California.
9. Botanical Influence on Illness.
   Second Edition Melvyn Werbach, third Line Press Tarzana, California. 2000.
10. Smart Fats.
    Michael Schmidt. Frog Publishing Berkeley, California.
11. Clinical Nutrition for Pain, Inflammation, and Tissue Healing.
    David R. Seamen. NutrAnalysis, Inc. Henderson, North Carolina. 1998.
12. Consumers Guide to Herbal Medicine.
    Steven B. Karch. Advanced Research Press. 1999. Hauppauge, New York.
13. Encyclopedia of Natural Medicine.
    M. Murray and J. Pizzorno. Publishing. Rocklin, California.
14. American Society for Clinical Nutrition, AMERICAN JOURNAL OF NUTRITION supplement to volume 53, no. 1, Jan. 1991.

15. Balch, JF, and Balch, PA, PRESCRITION FOR NURITIONAL HEALING, Avery Publ, Garden City, NY, 1990.

16. Baumgartner, TG, PARENTERAL MICRONUTRITION, Lyphomed, div. fujisawa, Inc. 1991.

17. Beasley, JD,THE BETREYAL OF HEALTH, Random House, NY,19991.

18. Bendich, A., and Chandra, RK, MICRONUTRIENTS AND IMMUNE FUNCTION, Annals of New York Academy of Sciences, vol.587.

19. Bloch, AS, NUTRITION MANAGEMENT OF THE CANCER PATIENT, Aspen publ., Rockville, MD, 1990.

20. BOIK, J, CANCER AND NATURAL MEDICINE, Oregon Medical Press, Princeton, MN, 1995.

21. Burns, JJ, etal, THIRD CONFERENCE ON VITAMIN C, Annals of New York Academy of Sciences (ph.212-838-0230), vol.498,1987, ISBN 0-89766-391-8.

22. CONGRESS OF United States, Office of Technology Assessment, UNCONVENTIONAL CANCER TREATMENT, U.S Government Printing Office, Washington, DC,1990.

23. Personal Nutrition, Marie. A. Boyle and Sara long 2007.

24. Diamond, WJ, ET AL., DEFINTIVE GUIDE TO CANCER, Future Medicine Publishing, Tiburon, CA, 1997.

25. Falcone R, COMPLETE GUIDE TO ALTERNATIVE CANCER THERAPIES, Citadel Press, NY, 1994.

26. Hendler, SS, THE DOCTORS VITAMIN AND MINERAL ENCYCLOPEDIA, Simon & Schuster, NY, 1994.

27. Jacobs, M., VITAMINS AND MINERALS IN THE PREVENTION AND TREATMENT OF CANCER, CRC Press, Boca Raton, FL, 1991.

28. Kaminski, MV, HYPERALIMENTATION, Marcel Dekker Press, NY, 1985.

29. Laidlaw, SA, and Swendseid, ME, VITAMINS AND CANCER PREVENTION, Wiley & Sons 1991.

30. Machlin, LJ, HANDBOOK OF VITAMINS, Marcel Dekker Press, NY, 1991.

31. Meyskens, FL, and Prasad, KN, MODULATION AND MEDIATION OF CANCER BY VITAMINS, S. Karger Publ., Basel, Switzerland, 1983.

32. Meyskens, FL, AND Prasad, KN, VITAMINS AND CANCER Humana Press, Clifton.

33. Moss, RW, QUESTIONING CHEMOTHERAPY, Equinox Press, Brooklyn, NY.

34. Murray, MT, ENCYCLOPEDIA OF NUTRITIONAL SUPPLEMENTS, Prima Publ., Rocklin, CA, 1996.

35. National Academy of Science, DIET, NUTRITION, AND CANCER, National Academy Press.

36. Nixon, DW, (ed.), CHEMOPREVENTION OF CANCER, CRC Press, Boca Raton, FL, 1995.

37. Nixon, DW, CANCER RECOVERY EATING PLAN, Random House, NY, 1994.

38. Passwater, RA, CANCER PREVENTION AND NUTRITIONAL THERAPIES, Keats publ., New Canaan, CT, 1983.

39. Pelton, R., et al., ALTERNATIVE IN CANCER THERAPY, Simon & Schuster, NY, 1994.

40. Poirier, LA, et al., ESSENTIAL NUTRIENTS IN CARCINOGENESIS, Plenum Press, NY, 1986.

41. Presad, KN, and Meyskens, ML, NUTRIENTS AND CANCER PREVENTION, Humana Press, Clifton, NJ, 1990.

44. Prasad, KN, VITAMINS AGAISNTS CANCER, Healing Arts Press, Rochester, VT, 1984.

43. Quillin, P., BEATING CANCER WITH NUTRITION, Nutrition Times Press, Tulsa, OK, 2001.

44. Quilin, P.(eds), ADJUVANT NUTRITION IN CANCER TREATMENT Cancer Treatment Research Foundation, Arlington Heights, IL 1994.

45. Simone, CB, CANCER AND NUTRITION, Avery Publ., Garden City, NY, 1992.

46. U.S. Dept. Health Services, SURGEON GENERAL'S REPORT ON NUTRITION AND HEALTH, U.S. Government Printing Office (ph. 800-336-4797), 1988.

47. Watson, RR, et al. (eds), NUTRITION AND CANCER PREVENTION, CRC Press, Boca Raton, FL, 1996.

48. Werbach, MR, NUTRITIONAL INFLUENCES ON ILLNESS, Third Line Press Tarzana, CA, 1987.

49. Willner, RE THE CANCER SOLUTION, Peltec Publ., Boca Raton, FL 1994.

50. Anderson, G., THE CANCER CONQUERER, Kansas City, Andrews & McMeel, 1988.

51. Leshan, L., CANCER AS A TURNING POINT.

52. Casarjian, R., FORGIVENESS: A BOLD CHOICE FOR A PEACEFUL HEART, New York, Bantam, 1992.

53. Borysenko, J., MINDING THE BODY, MENDING THE MIND, New York, Bantam, 1987.

INDEX

(A)

Acne   81
Acquire Immune Deficiency Syndrome
(Aids)   113
Aging   90
Alpha Linoleic (ALA)   41
Alcohol   55,63,64,65,69
Almonds   43, 49, 119
Anchories   41, 44
Anemia   110
Anemia prevention   110
Antioxidants   33
Antioxidants Substance   33
Antibiotics   81,144
Apples   16, 44, 160
Arthritis Prevention and Disorder   102
Asthma   104
Asthma Prevention   104
Avocados   43, 160
Avocado Seeds   160

(B)

Bad fats   39
Baked Beans   46, 60
Balanced diet   20, 69
Balancing your food choices   68
Bananas   158

Barley   161
Beans   53, 158, 164
Beta-carotene   33, 82
Bile Consumption   114
Binging   64, 65
Biotin   125
Bison Buffalo   15
Bitter Kola   165
Bran muffins   60
Breathing easy   86
Breast self exam   98
Broccoli   13, 53,156
Brown rice   164

(C)

Cabbage   155
Caffeine 58, 88,   146
Calories   25
Calorie dense food   27
Calcium   83, 126
Cancer   141
Carbonated beverages   146
Carrots   155
Cassava   165
Causes of hearth burn   146
Causes of high cholesterol   48
Cayenne pepper   17
Cereals   161

Certain habits 4
Chamomile 14
Cheese 39, 50
Cherries 151
Chili pepper 157
Chocolate 46, 146
Choice for low fat foods example 44
Choline 59
Cholesterol Imbalance 138
Choosing your daily diet 19
Chronic use of anti-inflammatory drugs 144
Chronic disorders 145
Cinnamon 16
Citrus fruits 16, 158
Coconut 162
Common killers of good looks and good health 3
Common tools for detecting breast cancer 98
Consumption of raw and rough food 106
Corn 161
Cranberries 14
Crisp bread 53

(D)

Dairy products 58
Dermatologist 92
Designing a balanced diet 22
Diabetes 149
Diabetes mellitus 149
Diets 18
Diet Soda 61
Dietary Thermogenesis 15

Difficulty in Urinating 142
Digestive Enzymes 36
Diseases of the kidney 129
Drinking alcohols on an empty stomach 65
Drinking enough water 67
Drinking green tea 139

(E)

Eat a well balanced diet 69
Eating habits 62
Eat meals on a table 63
Eating fish 143
Eating moderate portion of food 67
Eat more of fiber 74
Eating plenty of whole grains fruits and vegetables 67
Eating on the run 64
Eating too fast 65
Eating while working 65
Eating variety of nutrients dense food 67
Eating without water 65
Early signs of breast cancer in women 98
Enzymes 35
Essential fatty acid (EFA'S) 40
Essential nutrients 29
Essential nutrients during pregnancy 31
Exercise 48, 73,76, 79, 97, 141
Excessive alcohol 90, 129, 131, 145
Excessive hot and spicy foods 144
Excessive tea and coffee 144

Excessive use of anti-inflammatory drugs   145
Eye disorder prevention   108

(F)

Fats   38
Fat Soluble   123
Fish   14, 143, 159
Fish and Omega-3 fatty acids   49
Fish oil   102
Flour and flour made pasta   52
Folic acid   125
Foods containing Omega-3   41
Foods containing Omega-6   42
Foods containing omega-9   42
Food Enzymes   36
Foods that burn fat   15
Foods that make you look older   55
Foods that can make you look younger   56
Foods that can cause body Odor   58
Forget about your troubles   89
Free radicals   33, 90
Fried   58
Fruit juice   60

(G)

Gall bladder disorder and diet   114
Gall bladder disorder and prevention   114
Garbanzo beans   53
Garlic   79,118
Gender   138
Genetic predisposition   144

General advice on foods   42
Get a good night sleep   134
Ginger   164
Good eating habits   63
Good fats   40
Good foods   52
Good health and good living   1
Grape fruit   159
Grape and red wine prevention of aging   57
Green   164
Green beans   164
Green tea   79, 143
Guavas   151

Healthy diet   23, 142
Healthy foods and some risk factors   60
Healthy life style that can lead to Longevity   12
Heart disease   131
Heredity   96
High fat fast foods   47
High fat foods   46
Holy Basil   57
How to lose belly fat   73

(I)

Ice cream   39
Increased blood cholesterol level   131
Indigestion   144
Infection   76, 144
Infertility in women and men   116
Iron   83, 127
It is always better to start reasonably early   6

It is never too late to say yes
to change   9

(M)

(K)

Macronutrients   29
Maintain a healthy weight   67
Make changes gradually   68

Keep a regular sleeping pattern   88
Key causes of pre-mature aging   90
Kidney disorder and diet   99
Kiwi fruit   153
Kola   165
Kombucha tea   79

Malaria fever and diet   112
Malaria and Prevention   112
Mangoes   53, 158
Melon   53, 162
Metabolic enzymes   36
Micronutrients   29
Millet   162
Monounsaturated fats   40, 42

(L)

(N)

Lack of exercise and poor diet   3
Lack of exercise   96, 129, 131, 138, 149
Late night eating   64
Learn to take 10,000 steps per day   74
Learn to relax and ease your
stress   100
Lemon   14, 162
Life style   3
Limit alcohol to 1-2 drinks per day   63
Limit the consumption of caffeinated
beverages   85
Limit your intake of salt and nitrite
cured foods   67
Liver disorders and diet   100
Low fat milk or yogurt   23, 162
Low fat foods   44
Low fat salad dressing   60
Lowering our cholesterol level   49
Lutein   33
Lung disorder and diet   111
Lung disorder and Prevention   111
Lycopene   33

Nausea   133
Nutrients and essential nutrients   29
Nutrients dense foods   31
Nutrients that can make us look younger
than our age.   82

(O)

Oat bran   23, 49, 161
Oat meal, oat bran and high fiber
foods   49
Olive oil   44
Omega-3 (Linoleic acids)   41, 42
Omega-3 deficiencies   41
Omega-6 (Linoleic acid)   41
Omega-9 (Oleic acid)   42
Onions   47, 154
Osteoarthritis   102
Other tips to stop you getting sick   78
Other warning signs of stroke   138

Overeating   64

(P)

Packaged snack foods   39

Palm oil   39

Paw paw   157

Peanut butter   43

Peanut oil   42

Peas   163

Phosphorus   127

Pineapple   157

Plantain   163

Polyunsaturated fats   40, 42

Potatoes   53, 119, 162

Prevention of kidney disorders   99

Prevention of liver disorders   100

Prevention of typhoid Disorders   101

Prevention of arthritis   102

Prevention of Asthma   104

Prevention of tooth disorder   106

Prevention of eye disorder   108

Prevention of anemia   110

Prevention of lung disorder   111

Prevention of malaria   112

Prevention of Aids   113

Prevention of Gall bladder disorder   114

Prevention of thyroid disorder   115

Preventing hypertension   129

Preventing heart disease   131

Preventing heart attack   31

Preventing stroke   136

Preventing cancer   141

Preventing prostrate cancer   141

Preventing stomach ulcer   144

Preventing heart burn   146

Preventing diabetes   149

Prevention is always better that cure   7

Processed foods and junk foods   58

Protein bars   60

Pumpkin   163

(R)

Raspberry   163

Red meat   50

Red pepper   157

Reducing blood cholesterol and fat   48

Reduce but don't eliminate certain foods   67

Reduction In calorie consumption   73

Reduce your intake of foods high in saturated fat   95

Reduce your weight in relation to your height   95

Reduce your salt consumption   95

Regular and persistent eczema   98

Relax your body and mind   88

(S)

Sage   164

Salads   46

Sandwiches   47

Saturated fats   39, 55

Selenium   83

Silicon   128

Soups   51

Soybeans   161

Spinach   158

Starving yourself   65

Steps to changing bad eating habits   71

Stomach ulcer   144
Stroke   136
Sugar   55
Sweet potatoes   53, 164

(T)

Tangerines   164
Tea   56
Ten tips for an energizing life style   85
Ten ways to ease your tension   86
Thyroid disorder   115
Tips for a healthy looking skin   69
Tips to avoid premature aging   90
Tomatoes   23,157
Tooth disorders   106
Tran's fats   39
Trans partially hydrogenated oils   52
Trimethylamine   59
Try to give up smoking   70
Typhoid fever   101

(U)

Using food to ease stress   64

(V)

Vitamin A   31, 33, 81, 96, 123
Vitamin B1   123
Vitamin B2   123
Vitamin B3   124
Vitamin B5   124
Vitamin B6   124
Vitamin B12   125
Vitamin C   33, 83, 109, 125

Vitamin E   33, 34, 82, 109, 126
Vitamin K
Vitamins that give longevity and keep
you younger   123

(W)

Walnuts   42, 49
Water
Water Cress   84
Watermelon   53
Water Soluble   123

(Y)

You must get rid of refined grains for
whole grains   73

(Z)

Zinc   83, 127
Zollinger EllisonSyndrome   145